# Maintaining Control

# Maintaining Control

## An introduction to the effective management of violence and aggression

**Bob Willis** Cert Ed, 4th Dan (EKGB/WKSA), EKGB Coach,
Professional Defensive Tactics Trainer, Southport, UK

**John Gillett** ENMH, RNMH
1st Level Nurse, Alternative Futures, Liverpool, UK

A member of the Hodder Headline Group
LONDON

First published in Great Britain in 2003 by
Arnold, a member of the Hodder Headline Group,
338 Euston Road, London NW1 3BH

http://www.arnoldpublishers.com

Distributed in the United States of America by
Oxford University Press Inc.,
198 Madison Avenue, New York, NY10016
Oxford is a registered trademark of Oxford University Press

*British Library Cataloguing in Publication Data*
A catalogue record for this book is available from the British Library

*Library of Congress Cataloging-in-Publication Data*
A catalog record for this book is available from the Library of Congress

ISBN 0 340 81036 X

1 2 3 4 5 6 7 8 9 10

Commissioning Editor: Georgina Bentliff
Development Editor: Heather Smith
Project Editor: Anke Ueberberg
Production Controller: Lindsay Smith
Cover Design: Amina Dudhia

Typeset in 10pt Sabon by Pantek Arts Ltd, Maidstone, Kent
Printed and bound in Malta

What do you think about this book? Or any other Arnold title?
Please send your comments to feedback.arnold@hodder.co.uk

# CONTENTS

*About the authors*                                                vi
*Foreword*                                                         vii
*Acknowledgements*                                                 ix

**1** Introduction                                                 1
**2** Causative factors                                            8
**3** Awareness                                                    23
**4** Fear management and responses                                38
**5** Verbal confrontations and communication                     43
**6** Responsibility and accountability                            66
**7** Non-aversive breakaway techniques                            72
**8** Physical interventions                                       106
**9** Understanding and managing diverse behaviours                113
**10** Post-incident                                               116
**11** External risk management and personal safety                122

*Conclusion*                                                       136
*Additional information*                                           139
*References*                                                       140
*Index*                                                            143

# ABOUT THE AUTHORS

**Bob Willis** Cert Ed, 4th Dan (EKGB/WKSA), EKGB Coach.

Bob Willis is a former police defensive tactics trainer with more than 20 years' experience of both self-defence and traditional martial arts. In 1988 he established the acclaimed Personal Safety Promotion (PSP) system that has successfully introduced training courses in personal safety, aggression management and self-defence to hospitals, schools, universities and businesses across the UK.

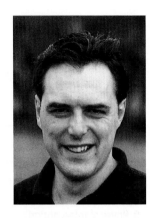

**John Gillett** ENMH, RNMH, NVQ Assessor.

John Gillett has worked professionally in the clinical environment since 1984, dealing extensively with clients who demonstrate severe challenging behaviour. He is also an experienced martial arts and long-standing PSP instructor, specializing in facilitating training courses in breakaway and intervention techniques for clinical application.

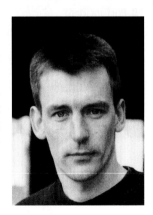

# FOREWORD

It is interesting to observe the changing demographic with respect to the victims of violence, in particular the reports of increases in aggressive and violent attacks on members of the clergy, who are now acquiring the skills of managing aggressive incidents to promote their personal safety. The British Dental Association has reported increasing levels of incidents and assaults upon dentists and dental staff. It seems that no individual or any organization that provides a service to people is immune to aggressive and violent incidents.

People, it has been said, have become more demanding and assertive. Expectations have increased and as a consequence this appears to be leading to increased potential for conflict situations. Each and every situation is unique and therefore it is impossible to provide instant solutions. Be prepared to discover that what may work in one situation, or with another person, may not work as well, or at all, on another occasion. It is a point worth remembering that no amount of skill or knowledge of techniques can provide for every event – sometimes nothing works. However, personal safety is the main concern and the techniques offered in this text will certainly assist you in dealing with this area of human conflict.

In order for people to deal with potential incidents, managers, services and organizations are investing in training programmes, as it has been found that staff who are trained, well-supported and confident in their work are more able to handle difficult situations effectively. The techniques and skills utilized in this book have been drawn from a number of areas where people are interacting in the delivery of services. This text is recommended to those who feel they have a need to acquire and develop more effective strategies, both to deal with potential conflict and to promote their personal safety.

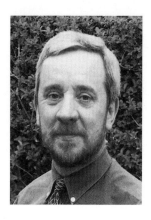

**John Greaves** Curriculum Advisor, BSc (Hons), ENMH, RNMH, RMN, RCNT, RNT, Cert Ed

# ACKNOWLEDGEMENTS

This text is an extension of a course module developed originally for the Personal Safety Promotion (PSP) project and the efforts of the PSP instructors involved in facilitating the sessions is recognized, in particular John Barnes, Linda Hindley, Hayley Fielden, Mike Fedyk, Dave Wilkins, Steve Rimmer, Rik Gillett, Rudi Elmquist, Derek Ridgway, Yvonne Lovelady, Andy Sharrock, George Gilbert, Lyndon Foster, Mike Phair, Mark Robinson, Ian Coleman, Kath Liversage and Jonathan Staples.

Thank you to all the hospitals, schools, colleges and businesses that have continued to use the PSP system, in particular John Greaves at the Edge Hill School of Health Studies and Gerry Drummy at John Moores University School of Health Studies.

Credit for the depth of expertise in practical technique goes to Steve Cattle, whose inspiration continues to motivate.

Special thanks to Jonathen Staples, Mark Standen, Paul Wright, Hayley Fielden, Liam Ainscough and Raj Patel for their assistance with this project.

Photography: Bob Willis, Stephanie Mann.

# Chapter 1

# INTRODUCTION

In modern society it is almost impossible to pass through a working day without some form of interaction with other individuals. Whether in a working or social capacity, for many people it is inevitable that they have some form of communication with clients, colleagues, service providers or the general public. Whenever there is interaction with others there is always the possibility, no matter how slight, that a confrontation may occur. Confrontations can be either verbal or physical, and individuals working in many occupations, particularly those working within the forces or in a clinical environment, may find themselves involved in an aggressive or violent situation.

Although it may be anticipated that serving police or prison officers will encounter a degree of violence as a part of their professions, it is less acknowledged that clinical professionals may equally be exposed to instances of extreme aggression. Professionals within law enforcement are likely be equipped with batons, CS sprays or possibly even some form of firearms. Beyond this they will receive introductory and ongoing training in self-defence and control techniques. Clinical professionals have no form of defensive weapon to come to their aid and receive little or no training in how to cope with violence or aggression.

In October 1998 the *Nursing Times*[1] published the results of a survey questioning almost 1000 individuals working in the medical profession in the UK. The findings revealed that 47 per cent of respondents had been physically assaulted in the previous year alone, whereas 85 per cent of respondents had been subjected to verbal abuse during the same period. Further to drawing on their own experience, 97 per cent of those surveyed knew a nurse who had been physically assaulted during the same year.

This survey highlighted a problem that the Department of Health (DoH) had previously targeted for improvement. A document released by the DoH in 1998 had already outlined its intention to 'stamp out violence and improve conditions'[2] within the NHS.

Despite a commitment to improve standards, it is not a problem that can be resolved quickly or easily.

Two years on from the survey and instances of violence within the NHS were still making headline news. In February 2000 nurse Alison Shortman was violently attacked in the grounds of Southmead Hospital at Bristol. Her assault was documented by journalist Richard Smith of the *Daily Mirror*, who quoted that staff at Southmead 'were in a state of terror – matching the nationwide mood of NHS workers'.[3] The same edition of the newspaper also reported on the assault of local GP, Dr Ian Brooman, in Swanley, Kent. Dr Brooman was savagely attacked by a knifeman in his own surgery, seemingly because, 'he refused to supply medication'.[4]

Smith's article reported that 50 per cent of working nurses had been physically assaulted and that 90 per cent of them had been subjected to verbal abuse. Even allowing for media sensationalism there was still a worrying number of cases cited, including casualty sister Theresa Ross, who reported four attacks in the same number of years. Concluding the article was the final figure of 65,000 violent attacks reported within the NHS during 1999 alone, two-thirds of them being aimed at nurses.

Little over a year later on 29 January 2001, the *Guardian*[5] again raised the issue of violence against NHS staff. Health correspondent, James Meikle, wrote of an average 500 violent incidents a year reported by each hospital across the UK, with one Trust claiming that complaints about violence had quadrupled. The newspaper article was compiled with information taken from a piece by Adam Geldman for the journal *Health Service Report* and went on to quote an average annual increase of 20 per cent in aggressive incidents across the NHS. However, the interest of the general media in violence within the health service concentrates solely on the NHS, it misses the unknown numbers of violent incidents within the private health care industry.

For both the NHS and private hospitals, as for any major employer, violence can lead to low morale and rising costs – through increased absenteeism, higher insurance premiums and compensation claims. The image of the establishment can also be tarnished, making it difficult to recruit and retain staff. Obviously, physical assaults are dangerous, but serious or persistent verbal abuse or threats can also damage employees' health through stress or anxiety. Smith's report in the *Daily Mirror*[3] claimed that almost half the nurses serving in the UK had considered leaving the profession.

These examples are only representative of a short period, covering a mere four years, but they do provide a clear indicator of an ongoing issue that has the potential to affect efficiency, service and, above all, the well-being of working professionals. Over time the trend for increased episodes of violence may be reversed, particularly if training is expanded and safety principles implemented, but the issue is unlikely to be eradicated.

Although the general media may not be considered as a pure source for referencing, it does provide an unsurpassed, straightforward insight into a high-profile issue that cannot be ignored and of which the general population is becoming increasingly aware. The year 2001 also saw the NHS issue a document through the Health Development Agency entitled *Violence and Aggression in General Practice. Guidance on Assessment and Management.* Intended to assist with guidance and management, its opening statement was: 'Acts of violence are a real threat in primary care. They may cause serious injury and working in an atmosphere of continuing threat is profoundly damaging to the confidence and morale of staff'.[6]

Clinical professionals dealing with mental health clients are often at an even greater risk than those working in general practice, a fact that has been well documented historically. In their manual aimed at nurses and health care workers, *Managing Violence and Aggression*, Mason and Chandley explored the relationship between mental health and violence, concluding: 'The idea of a relationship between violence and mental disorder has a long and chequered history. Most early accounts of mental aberration involve, to one degree or another, some aspect of violent behaviour occurring during phases of psychiatric crisis'.[7]

Citing the founder of modern psychoanalysis, Sigmund Freud, Mason and Chandley also identified that aggression is often a response to pain and frustration, and that the elements of the human mind are in conflict with each other, but the mental mechanisms in healthy individuals allow for resolution of these tensions. This principle alone clearly acknowledges the potential for aggression from mental health clients, with the authors further stating: 'just as the theory of homicidal monomania allowed 'dangerousness' to become the domain of psychiatry, so too did the developing theories of violence and aggression become medicalized concepts'.[7]

It is not just the clinical profession that is under fire, many other sectors have mounting problems to deal with. In a feature printed during March 2001, *The Times* led with the headline, 'I was attacked with a bottle, a knife and a baseball bat'.[8] Teachers, including lecturers in further and higher education, are also becoming targets, and yet there is no formal training to help them to manage aggression in the academic arena, whether from students or parents.

Although employers have a legal duty under the Health and Safety at Work Act 1974[9] to ensure, so far as is reasonably practicable, the health, safety and welfare at work of their employees, this often does not extend to protecting employees from assault. Responsibilities under the Act include employers providing a safe system of work and a safe working environment. Employees themselves have a responsibility to take reasonable care of themselves and other people who may be affected by their acts or omissions at work.

Beyond this, Article 5 of the European Convention for Human Rights 2000 outlines that everybody is entitled to 'the right to liberty and security of the person'.[10] Security of the person, by its nature, includes safety from physical assault or even intimidation.

Personnel training can be provided and procedures may be set in place to help reduce potential incidents or to manage them more professionally. Budgetary and time constraints may dictate that the required specialist training is either not viable or not convenient for some employers. However, for staff, a basic understanding of the principles of management of violence and aggression can help to ensure their personal safety if they become involved in a confrontation and can, in many instances, help to avoid the situation completely.

Effective management is always proactive. To be reactive when dealing with aggression management will always be too late and, consequently, an understanding of the subject is invaluable. Knowledge will not render anybody immune to attack and some confrontations may well prove unavoidable, but situations can be resolved positively with the correct skills. By simply having an increased sense of awareness many individuals may identify and diffuse potentially aggressive situations before they become a problem. Similarly, a more aware individual will respond more readily if under pressure.

When looking at the overall issue of safety, actual incidents are the least important point of focus. The environment, combined with awareness and attitude, can prove far more important to efficient management of situations. Should a confrontation occur, much may be learnt from studying the events leading up to the situation, along with the actions of those involved. Debriefing all those involved is also extremely important, but in many cases only the assault itself is analysed and nothing is either resolved or learnt.

Safety outside the traditional working environment is an issue that is more readily acknowledged as violent crime is increasingly documented in the media. Although statistically the chances of being assaulted remain relatively low, people need to be aware of the dangers and to be equipped with the skills and strategies to manage any potential threat realistically. Clinical professionals must also take seriously their safety when out in the community, in particular individuals making home visits, sometimes in remote areas and out of traditional working hours. A combination of concentrating on the task at hand, and working at a strange location or time of day, could lead to disorientation and vulnerability, particularly when working with unknown individuals.

Health authorities, clinical organizations and law enforcement agencies all have policies and training modules to cover the basics of dealing with violence and aggression. Countless other employers are also beginning to recognize their moral, as well as legal, responsibility to ensure the safety of their staff and clients who may be exposed to violence or aggression. However, the existing training material is often limited and subject to financial and logistical restrictions.

Effective aggression management is an issue of paramount importance in ensuring the safety of working professionals, and it should not be restricted or compromised through pressures from other factors. It is both controversial and complex in nature, and this text is intended only to provide an introductory insight to the subject, introducing the reader to a range of simple but proven strategies to assist in dealing with potential confrontations. The text is intended to be easily accessible but it is not a stand-alone package, having been structured to provide a basic insight or to complement the many training programmes that are currently in place.

The emphasis of this text is on personal safety, with the importance being placed on the integrity of the working professional. The techniques illustrated within the text are not intended as self-defence or 'control and restraint' moves; they are simply breakaway techniques, designed purely to assist individuals to remove themselves from a threatening situation. Accepting them as such and combining them with the theory principles also outlined within the text means that the concept of positive aggression management becomes more of an achievable reality.

Indeed, the subject of traditional control and restraint (C&R) is always changing and always contentious in nature. Some training providers have repackaged their programmes to the more politically friendly 'care and responsibility', using the same abbreviation applied to what is a very similar syllabus of techniques. A consultation document by Professor Kevin Gournay was issued in 2001 by the United Kingdom Central Council for Nursing, Midwifery and Health Visiting (UKCC) and reported that: 'there is a need to offer some clarification regarding the methods of physically intervening by use of breakaway and restraint techniques'.[11]

Although clarification may be needed, the document also confirms openly that:

> It seems clear that violence in in-patient settings is a considerable problem and it is obvious that staff in direct contact with patients are at risk. Furthermore, we must note that in-patients (and probably visitors) are also at significant risk of assault by other in-patients.[12]

The UKCC document analyses the history, usage and implications or consequences of applying C&R, but in the summary cannot avoid the issue that 'violence in the NHS is common and particularly so in mental health services'.[13] The importance of C&R as a vital tool is clearly acknowledged, but this overshadows the need for simple training in breakaway techniques and personal safety principles. There needs to be a clearer distinction made between the two practical disciplines, particularly in their application and their purpose.

Breakaways, such as those outlined within this text, are solely intended and employed to ensure personal safety in any circumstance, with full consideration to legal recourse being their underpinning principle. They are most valid when the user is alone or isolated and has no wish to control the aggressor, merely the need to escape successfully and to preserve their own integrity. Although reasonable consideration must always be given to the need for physical techniques, far more important is the management of oneself, practice, and the environment. This principle, supported by increased awareness and a basic grounding in breakaway techniques will combine to greatly reduce the risk of being injured or worse, whether inside or outside the working environment.

In orientation the following work may appear to be aimed solely at practitioners working in an inpatient setting, and primarily to those dealing with mental health issues and challenging behaviours. The reality, however, is that the principles and techniques enclosed are valid for anybody working in any clinical occupation, including general practitioners, paramedics, midwives and even management, reception and security personnel. Quite simply, the principles of the effective management of violence and aggression are relevant for anyone who has direct contact with others, whether professionally or socially.

# Chapter 2

# CAUSATIVE FACTORS

## INTRODUCTION

Almost all violent or aggressive incidents have one thing in common – a causative factor – or, put more simply, a reason for its occurrence. It is rare for violence to arise for absolutely no reason whatsoever, although often the reasons will not be readily identified. Even 'street' offenders, such as opportunist thieves, will have a prime motive to assault their victims, which is to ensure that they get what they want quickly in order to minimize the risk of capture. Similarly, other street crimes will often have easily recognizable motives for the use of aggression. Why violence happens within a working environment, especially within a clinical setting, is less easily understood, but it often occurs as a result of one of the following 'accelerators' or 'catalysts'.

The causative factors documented below do not form an exhaustive list, they are merely the most readily acknowledged, and explored so that they may be identified and more easily understood. If causes are understood, provision can be made to manage them using an informed and professional approach, recognizing relevant limitations and their possible effect on personal safety.

## COMMON CATALYSTS

### THE ENVIRONMENT

When new clients or visitors arrive at an organization or establishment they have certain expectations, which will normally include a desire for efficient and helpful service. Expectations may be destroyed immediately if the environment of an organization is below the standard anticipated. If a waiting area is dirty or in poor decorative order, visitors may well feel demeaned or uncared for. This can make them defensive instantly and may also result in difficult or aggressive behaviour. Similarly, a shortage of seating, or even uncomfortable chairs, could contribute to clients' negative impressions.

Creating a good impression undoubtedly contributes to a safer and more relaxed organizational environment. It is good practice to ensure that all the public areas of an establishment are clean and in a good state of decorative repair. Ideally, waiting areas or communal rooms should have reading material available and, if practicable, basic refreshment facilities. It is often thought that there is little point in providing a nice environment when clients appear not to respect it and are prone to destroy it. However, people are far more likely to respect an environment if it is in good condition to begin with.

A 'no smoking' policy will not be readily accepted by everybody but, equally, will win favour with others. Providing that everything else is of a high standard it is unlikely that this policy alone will create a major problem, but providing a smoking area as well will provide for all visitors' potential needs. Smokers may well become frustrated when not provided for, but non-smokers will also become agitated if exposed to tobacco fumes.

## THE ORGANIZATION

Many individuals do not find it easy to deal with a large organization and as a result they can sometimes feel alienated or even intimidated. They can perceive themselves as outsiders and the organization as cold, impenetrable and uncaring. This can automatically make them fearful and consequently defensive.

Communication with large organizations can sometimes seem to be dehumanized, particularly on the telephone, where people are constantly exposed to protracted automated answering systems that often negate any human interaction at all. If human contact is established, individuals may constantly be referred to different members of staff, sometimes without even knowing the names of those who may have dealt with them. This sort of protracted communication process can easily serve to confuse and frustrate. If the service-provider uses unfamiliar jargon or hides behind rules and policies, the notion of the insider against the outsider is enhanced – so placing clients at a greater feeling of disadvantage.

During a meeting the simplest way of breaking down the psychological barriers between individuals and the organization is to be as personable as possible. Being approachable, friendly and utilizing open gestures makes it easier for people to relax and helps to allay apprehension. Always use your name, ideally your full name or first name only, and attempt to convey a genuine interest in clients' problems and concerns. Taking notes and recording information can demonstrate visibly that you are taking a genuine interest in clients, as well as providing a record of the meeting that can be referred to during any subsequent contact.

Personal interaction, whether through telecommunications or, preferably, face-to-face, serves to break down any barriers to effective communication and reduces the gap between the organization and individuals.

## WAITING TIMES

As society moves at an ever faster pace people do not expect to have to wait, and they can often become increasingly frustrated when they have to do so. Having to wait for a long period of time is a critical factor in the fuelling of aggression. Should prolonged waiting times be unavoidable, appropriate facilities should be provided for clients, such as good seating, reading materials, refreshments and well-maintained toilet facilities. If children are involved then simple toys or drawing equipment can be made available in order to avoid them becoming bored or distracted. Whilst children themselves may not present a direct problem, their behaviour through boredom may irritate others or dictate that they need to be reprimanded, which their parents could resent.

An unfair queuing system is another potential catalyst to aggressive tension and therefore it is vital to ensure the fairest method possible is employed. The urgency of clients' needs will mean that some people will need to wait for longer than others, but in these instances a pleasant environment can serve to calm any impatience and enhance acceptance of the situation. As already stated, the environment plays a major part in controlling aggression when people have to wait and it needs to be as pleasant and well-equipped as organizational resources and imagination will permit. Fortunately, simple items such as magazines and basic toys can be obtained relatively cheaply but are invaluable in promoting a relaxed atmosphere.

## LACK OF INFORMATION

A common accelerator of aggression is found when individuals cannot readily obtain information about how to deal with their problems or how any treatment is progressing, whether it be their own or that of someone close to them. Lack of clear information leads to frustration, which in turn can lead to aggression. Clear information should be available to tell people what they need to know or where they may need to go and how best to get there.

If initial contact has been made but is not followed up, clients may feel that information is being kept from them deliberately or that the organization simply does not care about them. Organizations need to keep clients updated regularly about any ongoing cases, including making periodic courtesy calls, even when there may be no additional information available. Staff should never avoid speaking to clients and should never make up a response or pretend that they know the answers. It is far more prudent to be honest and admit to not having the relevant information or knowledge, but to then to offer to do something to find out.

## STAFF ATTITUDE

Not all people are suited to dealing directly with other individuals, but whereas a lack of knowledge can cause resentment, the way in which verbal information is delivered may also create frustration. Being pleasant and courteous promotes a sense of good will. Adopting an impersonal or abrupt manner when dealing with others will almost certainly prompt some form of negative response in return. Similarly, appearing disinterested will undoubtedly fuel tension.

Certain situations may require regular contact, which, if it proves to be below the clients' anticipated standards, will have a cumulative effect resulting in resentment, tension and frustration – all of which are catalysts for aggression.

Employees in positions of responsibility or authority who adopt a superior manner over their staff and/or clients are likely to breed resentment and potential aggression. Successful people management is structured upon numerous skills, including decisiveness, fairness, integrity, being approachable, and the ability to communicate effectively and confidently at all levels, but far more importantly, a genuine interest in their staff along with a willingness to praise and not to patronize or demean.

## CAUSATIVE FACTORS – SUMMARY

- The environment.
- The organization.
- Waiting times.
- Lack of information.
- Staff attitude.

Most of the causative factors outlined above can lead to aggression through frustration. Although these reasons are generally accepted as prime accelerators for violence or aggression within the workplace, there are a number of other causative factors which will affect service-providers within certain areas of clinical practice. Individuals who work with mental health issues or with clients who exhibit some form of challenging behaviour may anticipate having to cope with some instances of aggressive behaviour.

Individuals most likely to demonstrate challenging behaviour include those with learning difficulties or with mental health problems. In many instances, people with learning difficulties will use relatively unco-ordinated types of attacks, such as grabbing or hair pulls. Sometimes individuals with restricted motor skills may not communicate their needs adequately and can also strike out in frustration or rage.

Clients with mental health problems may use varying degrees of aggression, but in some instances will still be able to demonstrate sharp cognitive processes and good motor skills, which when combined will enable planned or premeditated attacks. Again, this is something that needs to be considered.

Not all people with challenging behaviours are in residential care and there is always a possibility of an aggressive encounter in any environment. Semi-residential care and concepts such as 'care in the community' have seen numerous clients reintegrated back into society, in some cases prematurely, and there are many other individuals who have never even been in care. Whether encountered on the ward, in the street or in any other situation, it is important to understand the causes of challenging behaviour.

## Case study 2.1

*Background*
Charlie* is a 34-year-old man who has a learning disability as a result of contracting meningitis at the age of 13 weeks. As a result of damage to the brain, Charlie also suffers from temporal lobe epilepsy. His treatment as a child involved anticonvulsant medication, which may have induced a schizoid affective disorder as he matured. There is no concrete evidence of this; however, there are many indications to suggest that the treatment at such an early age may have made the situation worse. Charlie also developed a hearing deficit as a result of the damage his brain received from the illness.

▶

Charlie's childhood could be considered as traumatic. His mother found that because of his increasing temper tantrums and aggression she could not cope alone. Charlie was sent to a school for the deaf, initially from Monday to Friday, and coming home at weekends.

As Charlie grew older and stronger his aggression became more apparent. A lot of issues arose from communication difficulties, partly from his delayed development and, more likely, from his auditory deficit.

As time progressed, service-providers also found that they had difficulty in providing for Charlie's complex needs, and as a result, he was moved from one care setting to another, ultimately ending up in a large mental institution on an assessment unit.

Charlie was eventually found a placement in a small secure unit for people with similar needs, where he still lives today.

### The present

Charlie can become quite violent for no apparent reason. However, there is always a reason for this. One moment Charlie may appear happy and content, and then suddenly erupt into such a rage that he will attack the nearest person, often someone he likes, by punching, kicking and grabbing. Proactive and reactive strategies, based upon the experience of those working with Charlie, are in place as guidelines for this situation. Unfortunately, the proactive measures do not always work as Charlie has already lost his temper by this stage.

Staff working with Charlie are trained in the management of aggression, which includes many sub-issues, such as values, awareness, mental illness and individual care, all of which contribute to an holistic approach when planning care.

Over the years, Charlie has learnt ways of coping with his anger, though at a very simple level. For example, if he is simply in a bad mood he will spit at the nearest person and leave, going to sit quietly in his private room.

If Charlie wants or needs something and cannot ask, or will not do so, he may sit and brood about the issue, sometimes resulting in aggression. This is usually the point where staff need to be very aware; it may simply be enough to ask Charlie if he wants something, to which he will usually reply, for example, *'tea'*, *'sandwich'* or perhaps request a walk to the shop.

Everyday interactions are very important to Charlie, whether it be body language, speech or general appearance in mood. With such complex needs it is important to recognize that problems will arise on a regular basis, but risk may be minimized by forward planning, assertiveness, teamwork and, above all, compassion and true commitment to fellow human beings.

*\*Permission has been given to document this case study. 'Charlie' is a pseudonym.*

## SPECIFIC 'CLINICAL' CAUSES OR CATALYSTS

### DISORIENTATION

Aggression may be caused as a result of disorientation, including reduced memory, concentration or attention, owing to organic mental disorders. People with learning difficulties may fail to understand what is required of them, particularly if those speaking to them use complex grammar. Shouting at clients can worsen the situation, as they may well recognize that they have done something wrong but will not necessarily know exactly what.

In order to prevent individuals from becoming confused and/or frightened, it is good practice to speak slowly and concisely, using simple words and short sentences. Similarly, open gestures and friendly body language, including smiling, will help to ease any tension created by disorientation.

### INABILITY TO COMMUNICATE

Many individuals with mental health problems and learning difficulties find it extremely hard to communicate their needs. Understanding this problem will not necessarily stop these individuals from becoming frustrated, or even violent, but it will ultimately ensure more tolerance and enable care plans to be structured for them.

Having accepted that there may be a communication issue it is good practice to give clients time to express themselves and to make time to listen to them. Rushing individuals will only heighten their frustration, whereas taking the time to try to understand their needs will serve to calm and build a more productive relationship.

### CHANGES IN MEDICATION

Although it is often necessary to alter routinely clients' medication, doing so can cause a number of behavioural side-effects. It is not uncommon for clients to know what their medication is for and to be familiar with its results, but should it change they can easily become confused or excited. If new medication is given it may result in some form of behavioural side-effect or symptom, such as depression or elation. Some clients may not be able to understand this themselves, and may become frightened or confused, which in turn could lead to aggression.

## THE ENVIRONMENT

Whereas a poor environment is a recognized accelerator of aggression, this situation may be significantly worsened for those with learning disabilities or mental health problems, where perception may be distorted. These individuals, too, may be concerned about the decorative order of the establishment, but will also probably be more sensitive to basic elements, such as heat, light and noise. Equally, if clients already struggle to communicate they may well find it hard to express the fact that they are too hot, or too cold, or cannot tolerate the noise.

Each individual may respond differently to various elements and consequently it may prove difficult to maintain an environment that is ideal for everyone, but it should be recognized that people are more likely to respond adversely to extremes of light and heat. Good management of the environment can work to limit the number of potential problems.

In extreme cases the size and layout of a room may prompt a violent episode from clients. Some people will insist on having more personal space than others, or they simply must have the room laid out exactly as they want it. If their desires are not met, this too can create problems. In their own room it is good to promote clients' autonomy and personal choice and to let them express themselves as they wish, so far as safety permits. Allowing freedom enhances well-being and this is usually then reflected in behaviour. It is more difficult in communal areas where several strong-willed individuals may gather, but with careful consideration and planning a compromise can usually be worked out, especially if clients have their own rooms exactly how they want them.

Thought must also be given to what exactly is in each room. Items such as kitchen utensils and glassware can readily be used as weapons, and similarly, large heavy objects, such as televisions, may be thrown during violent episodes.

It is accepted that it is not always possible or practical to use all safe items or to secure everything that could be picked up and thrown. Positive risk management requires a considered assessment of all areas within the establishment, with appropriate steps being taken to minimize or eradicate the use of potentially harmful items. Large objects, such as televisions, can be secured, whereas glassware and cutlery may be substituted by plastic products, or at the very least need to be monitored and possibly pieces issued and accounted for individually.

## PAIN

Pain is a barrier to effective communication and those in pain are often unable to communicate normally. When in pain people may behave in an uncharacteristic way and become aggressive, possibly due to an inability to cope with that pain or to communicate that they are in pain, or indeed that they may have an injury or illness. Aggression in these instances is borne from the pain itself and the resulting frustration or confusion. To regain control the priority must be to relieve the pain.

In extreme instances, aggression may not subside until pain is alleviated, forcing treatment to become a priority. In this situation, treatment or pain relief may need to be administered by a team. It would not be advisable for an individual to try and treat an aggressive client on a one-to-one basis.

## POSITIVE PSYCHOTIC SYMPTOMS

Some clients with mental health problems may suffer from delusional thoughts or exhibit a distorted sense of reality. This can include hearing voices, which may tell them to do something violent or aggressive, including self-harm. Similarly, the voices may tell them that something or someone else may be trying to harm or kill them. Both of these false beliefs can lead to aggression.

It is important when attempting to communicate with somebody exhibiting delusional behaviour that the practitioner speaks slowly and clearly in front of the client. Although it is recommended to have a number of staff available, only one person should attempt to communicate, as a mixture of voices may serve to heighten the false belief. Equally, radios, televisions and other such audible transmitters should be switched off to lessen any confusion.

## OBSESSIONS

Obsessions are unwanted thoughts, often concerning specific objects or individuals, prompting clients to act in a certain way. The subject may well realize that the rumination is silly, but simply cannot help acting upon it. Whilst violence is not always directly linked to such obsessions, in some instances clients may feel an overwhelming need to destroy the subject of their fixation and this can potentially lead to aggression. Clients' environments need to be managed proactively to avoid them coming into any unplanned contact with the subject of their obsession.

## INACTIVITY

When people are inactive they have more time to focus on their problems, which in turn can prompt challenging behaviour. When people are occupied they do not have time to dwell on their problems and instances of aggressive behaviour decrease. By providing a range of appropriate activities clients' energies may be channelled more positively. When inactive, people can also become bored and, as a result, may also become violent or aggressive.

## CHANGE

Certain clients will not respond well to change. Routine helps them to understand and to manage themselves, whereas changes lead to confusion, fear and distress, which in turn can result in violent or aggressive outbursts. In such instances it is prudent to limit any unnecessary change for clients.

## SPECIFIC CATALYSTS – SUMMARY

- Confusion.
- Inability to communicate.
- Changes in medication.
- The environment.
- Pain.
- Delusions.
- Obsessions.
- Inactivity.
- Change.

In the instance of a residential or 'known' client, all the above catalysts and causative factors may be managed to some extent through the use of care plans and proactive management of both staff and resources. However, there will always be new clients to deal with, who may well present new and unknown problems. By establishing a safe and relaxed environment, operated by well-trained and confident staff, it is possible to cater for most events.

## EXTERNAL CATALYSTS AND MOTIVES

In simple everyday terms there are more basic and readily identifiable motives for an attack outside the working environment.

Practitioners who work in the field, attending home visits or travelling extensively between different centres, may need to give closer consideration to their personal safety outside normally anticipated circumstances.

Although all the causative factors and catalysts may also contribute to a physical or verbal attack outside the traditional working environment, it is more likely to be a complete stranger, with a specific motive, who will confront somebody in the street. These types of assaults are often pre-planned by the aggressor and the victim will normally be totally unprepared for what happens. Assaults of this nature could happen at any location, at any time, and it is therefore difficult to manage or prepare for them. When the confrontation is over, it is unlikely that victims will ever see their attackers again or that there will be any trace of them. The basic motives for this situation are detailed below.

## PERSONAL GAIN

The most common motive for a personal attack in the street is that of personal gain, which normally takes the form of 'mugging' or similar opportunistic theft. If an assailant confronts someone in the street, the victim should strive at all costs to escape. Should this not be possible then target subjects have one of two choices: they can either give aggressors what they want or they can stand and fight to maintain possession of their property.

In a street situation it is advisable to give aggressors what they want in terms of personal possessions. For the sake of money, a bag or jewellery, which could well be insured, victims could potentially end up in hospital, or worse. It should be understood that personal belongings can be replaced, a human life cannot.

If surrendering personal possessions it is a good strategy to throw them as far beyond the aggressor as possible, shouting clearly, '*Here, take it!*' before pulling away and fleeing in the opposite direction while still shouting loudly for help. Having been discarded, the valuables will be lying still and quiet, whilst the victim is running away noisily. Research by the police in the United States has shown that aggressors will normally only ever pursue the valuables.

Should the victim merely hand over the possessions compliantly, the thief may well ask for further items, such as watches or rings. If the aggressor is male and the victim female then this may start a 'path of compliancy', which may lead to a more serious type of assault.

Many individuals refuse on principle to surrender their posses-sions, including even items that do not belong personally to them but to their employer. Although it is not desirable merely to surrender, a refusal will mean the aggressor will have to take the items they want, probably by means of force. The defender may not be in a position to win, particularly if the assailant has a weapon or an accomplice.

Practitioners making home visits may be considered as opportune targets by prospective thieves, who may believe them to be carrying medication or valuable equipment. There is an ethical dilemma when surrendering a medical bag, but ultimately practitioners will rarely be in a strong position to defend themselves against an unexpected inter-ception and they therefore may have little alternative but to relinquish a medical bag. Should practitioners suffer serious injury whilst trying to hold on to a bag they will probably lose it regardless, but will then be in no position to take care of themselves or anyone else.

## MALICE

Malicious attacks may be carried out by a known person with a spe-cific agenda, but may also be instigated by a complete stranger. These assaults can be premeditated or spontaneous and have no other motive than to inflict pain or suffering on the victim. Easily acknowledged examples of malicious attacks are revenge assaults and a variety of prejudices, including racial, religious and, in a grow-ing number of instances, even sporting rivalry.

## SEXUAL ASSAULTS

Home Office statistics released in the year 2000 reported that, on average, 6000 rapes and a further 17,500 indecent assaults were recorded by the police annually during the 1990s. The media in the UK at that time highlighted the report and exposed an official 'grey' figure, identifying that up to another 300,000 sexual assaults per annum were unrecorded.[14] Nigel Morris, reporting for the *Daily Mirror*, isolated data from the Home Office report that only between 10 per cent and 25 per cent of such crimes were actually reported.

With such statistics to be considered it should also be recognized that professional personal safety training cannot be taken lightly, or dismissed out of hand. Increased awareness, combined with good personal safety management, may significantly reduce exposure to situations likely to leave individuals vulnerable. These principles are outlined further in Chapter 11 and, if applied and then combined with more mainstream methods of self-defence, individuals will be provided with a base from which to manage better, or ideally avoid, assaults of this nature.

## IRRATIONALITY

Although personal gain, malicious and sexually motivated assaults appear to have motives that are recognized instantly, there are assaults that seem to have no motivating factor or reason behind them. In truth, this is rarely the case and on closer consideration the driving force behind the assault may be identified.

### Alcohol and drugs

More basic than aggressive or challenging behaviour, an irrational attack may commonly be inflicted by someone who may be under the influence of alcohol or drugs, prescribed or otherwise. Drugs and alcohol work effectively in lowering people's inhibitions, increasing their confidence and distorting their perceptions. In some instances this can cause individuals to behave in an illogical or aggressive manner.

An extreme example of this behaviour can also manifest itself as 'acute behavioural disturbance', which is often identified by bizarre behaviour, extreme aggression and excessive physical strength, combined with an apparent immunity to pain. This state can be brought on by the use of alcohol, drugs or as a result of a specific mental health problem. Other specific causes of acute behavioural disturbance include head injury, tumour, delirium and endocrine disorders.

This condition is classed as a medical emergency but caution must be exercised if attempting to restrain individuals, although this may prove necessary should they attempt to harm themselves or others. The methods used for restraint need to be considered carefully. Techniques should be approved, ethical and applicable. They should only be employed by personnel with the necessary skills and experience.

Some individuals may have another underlying problem that affects their behaviour, such as either a recognized learning difficulty or a specific mental health problem. Practitioners who deal with mental health issues can understand the problems experienced by these clients and the behavioural characteristics their condition may create. People who do not work in such an occupation will not recognize the symptoms for what they are and, to them, the behaviour might simply be classed as irrational.

In all instances, whether stimulus-prompted aggression or behavioural aggression, an assault will often appear to be totally and completely without motive to the victim, and in some instances, to the instigator once the event has passed.

## EXTERNAL MOTIVES – SUMMARY

* Personal gain.
* Malice.
* Sexual assault.
* Irrationality.

The four basic external motives are not issues for aggression management, and strategies for handling them come under personal safety studies as outlined further in Chapter 11. However, they are undoubtedly linked and there will always be areas of cross-over. The reality is that any individual could fall victim to an attack, borne from any of the catalysts and causative factors described, including the four prime external motives, whether at work or anywhere else. The chances are variable but the possibility is there.

Again, how to manage individual scenarios is best covered within the parameters of a personal safety course, but a very simple strategy for people to remember is that in a violent situation the less time they spend with the aggressor the less chance of them coming to harm. The exception and reality is that many clinical professionals have a duty of care to spend lengthy periods of time with patients who constantly pose a threat of violence. In such instances careful management of the environment, increased awareness, quality training and professional practice can limit the potential threat.

Should a situation, either in the workplace or externally, become too difficult or too violent to manage then it is always advisable to withdraw, by use of breakaway techniques if necessary. No one should ever attempt to deal with violence alone if help is near at hand or can be summoned. If help is unavailable then serious consideration must be given before attempting to manage the situation and the principles of the conflict resolution plan applied (see Chapter 3, 'Awareness').

Every person has their own beliefs, which will have been formulated as a result of their life experiences. These beliefs will often dictate their behaviour and responses in various situations. How they react in conversation and their perception of others will also be heavily influenced by these beliefs.

In the workplace service-providers must remain impartial and not let their own opinions and ideas influence or prejudice their actions and their work. Whilst being impartial they must acknowledge and try to understand the beliefs of others, even if they do not agree with them, and avoid creating a clash that could lead to a confrontation. Individuals' beliefs may also affect their responses to a violent or aggressive episode. Situations need to be managed without any pre-determined opinions or prejudices that could lead to excessive force or punishment being used. Maintaining control and preserving personal integrity is achievable by remaining professional, calm and impartial, regardless of the cause or nature of an incident.

# Chapter 3

# AWARENESS

## INTRODUCTION

A key element of the successful management of violence and aggression is a basic understanding of the principles of 'awareness'.

If individuals have a good general state of awareness, of themselves and their surroundings, the chances of them finding themselves involved in an aggressive confrontation are reduced. Many people do not pay a great deal of attention to their surroundings and to other people within the proximity. These individuals are not in a strong position to manage the environment or to pre-empt or contain any situation that may arise.

Increased awareness of self and surroundings are the first steps towards avoiding potential problems, but the subject encompasses much more than this, it includes an understanding of personal safety, crime prevention and, to a degree, common sense. In the instance of an actual assault, individuals would not reasonably be prepared to defend themselves if they were not aware of their attacker's presence.

Being aware of the surroundings within the workplace is a form of proactive management that can make the difference between prompting a confrontation or relaxing a potential aggressor. Having established that the environment can be a catalyst for violence and aggression, it should be maintained to the highest possible standard and all amenities kept in good order. Poor surroundings may be an indicator that service-providers are either not aware or that they simply may not care.

Certain environmental factors can contribute to the risk of a violent incident occurring. Simple things, such as the choice of colour scheme, can have a dramatic effect on some individuals. A subdued colour scheme may well be less provocative than a more dramatic choice. Poor visibility or accessibility can also prove contributory factors that can compromise safety within the workspace and also impede escape or intervention in an emergency.

Taking a few moments to appraise and amend the layout of a room can make a considerable difference to its effect on clients and to its practicality in function. If there is a reception area, it should not be isolated or removed from contact with the remainder of the establishment. A final consideration should be whether any furniture, fittings, accessories or ornaments could be used as potential weapons.

All public areas should be user-friendly, but easily managed, something that falls into the domain of risk management. Good, clean facilities should be provided and the surroundings made relaxing and safe. Pictures and plants enhance the locale but could easily be thrown as projectiles, dictating that they should be secured if reasonably possible to do so.

In large capacity units, such as Casualty departments, the use of security staff or even CCTV cameras may prove a practical deterrent, but they should not be used on wards or in general units, where client privacy is of consideration. Alarm systems linked by strategically located panic buttons are a more acceptable alternative, but often costly to install. The use of personal attack alarms, issued to each member of staff, may well prove a realistic compromise.

In some instances staff could come into contact with individuals who are known to be aggressive or violent, and indeed, as a part of their role others will be directly responsible for providing care for such clients. Policy may dictate that they cannot refuse service or care to such individuals, but provision must be made to deal with them safely.

It is possible that certain clients may have highly sensitive issues or problems that need to be dealt with. These people may well be upset or under stress and consequently exhibit behaviour that is out of character, such as weeping, shouting and physical violence. Being aware of potentially sensitive or problematic individuals, and more importantly, being aware of the specifics, will help to contain their behaviour. Being knowledgeable about the case and aware of any previous behavioural issues, and their outcome, will provide a solid basis to manage a situation. Not having the correct information will not only place an employee at a disadvantage but may also provoke an attack due to the client feeling uncared for or depersonalized.

Awareness of the environment, and of the people who enter it, is the crux of the effective management of aggression. Where practicable in a clinical situation, all clients should have appropriate and up-to-date care plans, which must take into consideration all medication and any tendencies to challenging behaviour. These care plans need to be strictly adhered to, and updated or amended as necessary, with all staff involved being notified accordingly. Having established safe surroundings and the specific requirements of individuals, it is then important to be aware of exactly what is happening at any given time.

## THE COLOUR CODE OF AWARENESS

An individual's degree of awareness is not something that is readily measurable. However, there is a colour code that may be used to identify an individual's condition of awareness and that provides a scale by which service-providers may assess their own potential for managing an aggressive encounter.

The colour code is a concept originally pioneered by the US Marine Corps during World War II and later refined by Colonel Jeff Cooper. It is a system that has since been used by numerous agencies, and is a proven method of managing self-awareness with respect to any potential confrontation situation.

There are five separate levels of awareness, each represented by a different colour. The first level is condition 'white'. At this level, individuals are totally unaware of anything that may be happening around them. They may be completely engrossed in their work, or in conversation. They may simply be relaxed, possibly even daydreaming. They are not aware of what is going on around them or of any people within their immediate vicinity. Should somebody become aggressive it is unlikely that the individual will be able to respond swiftly enough to manage the incident effectively.

The next level is 'yellow'. This is a state of relaxed awareness, where individuals are taking in everything that may be going on around them, even though they may be working or conversing. They are not so engrossed in their tasks that they become oblivious to, or detached from, their surroundings. They will not necessarily be expecting any problems, but are merely aware that things can change readily and need to be monitored.

'Orange' is a degree of alertness, when individuals have possibly identified a potential problem or threat. Something may have occurred to prompt this condition, although the exact nature of the threat may not be determined as yet. Prompts may include the arrival of somebody in the vicinity, or a change in behaviour of somebody already within the area. At this level, individuals are ready to take some form of appropriate action, which could include summoning assistance or identifying a potential escape route.

When the threat becomes real, individuals will reach condition 'red' – 'fight or flight' decision time. They are prepared to take whatever steps are necessary to manage the situation or, in extreme instances, to ensure their own personal safety. Their response may be to intervene, to defend or to flee. Escape may be made at this time using the routes identified whilst at condition 'orange'. At work, the two main options to consider are either to attempt to diffuse the situation or, if the threat is severe enough and there is no assistance available, to withdraw.

'Black' is the last level of the code and is the one condition that effective management should ensure is never actually reached. Neither escape nor containment have proved possible and the individual is under attack, either physical or verbal, and must do whatever is ethically necessary, with consideration to their duty of care to the client, in order to regain control and/or escape.

The colour code is a simple way to sum up individuals' awareness and may be applied to the workplace or even everyday life. To manage any situation successfully, service-providers must condition themselves to work constantly at condition 'yellow'. If they ever allow themselves to operate at the 'white' level, they will always be reacting and will not be in any position to manage a potential confrontation situation. Reacting to a situation is always going to be too late. The colour code is a proactive management method that can be readily adopted to ensure personal safety and effective management. Individuals at condition 'yellow' will be more perceptive, observant and more likely to 'read' situations successfully. Working at condition 'yellow' minimizes the risk of ever reaching condition 'black'.

## THE COLOUR CODE OF AWARENESS – SUMMARY

- White – subject relaxed or distracted – unaware.
- Yellow – relaxed awareness – observant.
- Orange – alertness due to stimuli – ready.
- Red – situation identified – decision time.
- Black – avoidance unavoidable – action.

Service-providers need to work constantly at condition 'yellow' to avoid reaching condition 'black' and must never be at condition 'white'.

## ASSERTIVE OR AGGRESSIVE?

Although an argument may be distressing, it is very easy for it to escalate into a physical assault. It is important to exercise caution in what is said, and exactly how it is said. Up to 93 per cent of all communication is through body language. It is often not what is said that creates a problem, but how it is said. Caution should be exercised during any verbal interaction. Words need to be selected carefully and any potentially provocative statements, expressions or gestures avoided.

Should a meeting or an interview become heated, it should be terminated immediately, by use of as much diplomacy as possible (see Chapter 5, 'Communication'). A common guideline in self-defence is that the less time spent with the aggressor, the less chance the defender has of becoming a victim. This is not always applicable within a care environment because of the needs and safety of clients. Quite simply, service-providers have a duty of care to clients, but this should not leave them exposed to danger. Being aware of self and environment, and managing both proactively, will lessen the risk potential to the staff in a conflict situation.

Body language is an important tool (see Chapter 5, 'Communication') but service-providers need to be aware of the signals they are transmitting. Their composure and posture, combined with the pitch and tone of their voices, can have a considerable impact on other individuals and may make the difference between a situation escalating or not. Having an assertive and confident manner will help maintain control of the situation, provided it is not overly so.

Being overassertive, or even aggressive, will often only serve to fuel a negative situation. It is important to understand and accept the basic difference between aggressiveness and assertiveness. A definition of *aggressive* is 'quarrelsome or belligerent',[15] which if accepted will undoubtedly lead to aggression and conflict. *Assertive*, however, may be defined as 'to put oneself forward in an insistent manner'.[16] By adopting more specific psychiatric definitions we understand that assertiveness is usually considered as normal, whereas aggression is often deemed abnormal, sometimes in degree, or even owing to pathological causes.

Assertive individuals strive to maintain control of a situation whilst considering the effect of their actions on colleagues, clients and the environment. Assertiveness does not necessarily negate being approachable, friendly or constructive. Those who adopt an aggressive approach will often merely push forward for what they want, with little or no consideration of others or consequences. Aggressive behaviour is a barrier to communication and a catalyst for further aggression. Logically, service-providers should strive to be assertive, achieving the necessary management decisions or strategy while being aware of their impact on others and amending their methods if necessary.

If service-providers are neither assertive nor aggressive in their practice, they may be exhibiting a passive nature. A definition of *passive* is 'not acting',[17] or even 'submissive'. A person working in a face-to-face role, particularly when dealing with potentially difficult or aggressive clients, is unlikely to operate effectively and manage efficiently if he or she is passive in nature.

The definitions are concise, but they do not begin to explore the individual character traits they attempt to describe. However, if it is accepted that people will behave in a certain manner then logic indicates that they should strive to be assertive if dealing with others in situations where conflict is a possibility.

## TEAM MECHANICS

Not only is the practitioner's personal attitude of the utmost importance, so is that of his or her colleagues. If working as part of a team, it is clearly productive if that team works together, adopting the same attitudes and principles, thus creating a level of consistency for clients.

Whilst people will always be different, owing to their own experiences, attitudes and belief systems, it is necessary for workers to establish a collectively productive environment. In some instances staff will readily connect with one another and good team mechanics are established naturally, whereas in others this can take time to happen and sometimes may never do so.

If there is a staff member who is aggressive in nature, this attitude will undermine the team working relationship, causing potential friction between staff. This situation is often recognized by clients and causes them to become unsettled also. Equally, an aggressive member of staff may fuel a negative response from clients or possibly other staff members, resulting in an aggressive incident. It should also be considered that some clients can become unsettled by an aggressive team member, and subsequently take out their aggression on another client, or an entirely different member of staff, possibly even at a later time.

## USING AWARENESS PRINCIPLES

During any interaction it is important to consider the other person's position or problem. Using open arm gestures while maintaining good eye contact will help to reassure clients of a genuine interest. Looking downwards or dipping the head may be interpreted as either hiding something or as vulnerability. Similarly, looking to either side may be perceived as disinterest, or possibly even bore-dom. For a potential aggressor these are 'go' signals. Service-providers need to be aware of their own body language so that they appear assertive, using confident and positive gestures to help take control of the situation.

It is important also to observe the other person's body language in order to determine whether or not they are preparing a physical attack. Clenched fists are clearly a hostile gesture, as is prolonged eye contact, and indicate that a person may be preparing to attack.

Awareness of self and surroundings will allow individuals to manage a situation, but when an actual confrontation occurs, which is sometimes unavoidable regardless of any proactive management strategies, it is vital that only an appropriate and ethical response is used. The degree of response necessary will relate directly to the potential threat, or more importantly, the individual's perception of the potential threat.

A good guideline for consideration when measuring a relevant response is a 'conflict resolution plan', which is structured to weigh up all the relevant factors and designed to help rationalize an appro-priate response. Although individuals will not pause in the heat of an attack to try to remember the plan, it is worthy of consideration so that the principles of appropriate response are understood.

## CONFLICT RESOLUTION PLAN

Conflict resolution systems are widely used by police forces and other agencies to enable personnel to better manage any potential conflict. The proven principles facilitate reasoned assessment and a reasoned response to an aggressive situation.

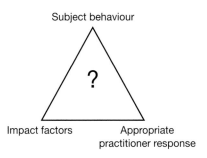

**Figure 3.1** Conflict resolution plan.

The three corners of the triangle relate to the three factors that will determine what course of action should be taken, and to what level. The question mark in the centre merely identifies where all three factors meet to give the relevant necessary response, which remains unknown until the other three points are considered.

## SUBJECT BEHAVIOUR

Subjects' behaviour is the first point for consideration. Clients may be compliant, in which case the mere presence of the practitioner could well prove enough to end any situation, or at the other extreme, they may be physically violent, in which case defensive techniques, and possibly even control techniques, may be necessary.

Any response should be directly appropriate to the level of threat and the intensity of behaviour exhibited. If clients were compliant it would be excessive to meet that level of confrontation with physical intervention or practical defence techniques. Equally, if they were extremely violent, the use of verbal communication may not resolve the problem.

Table 3.1 relates to the first two corners of the triangle and identifies common behaviours and suggests appropriate responses to that measured behaviour. There should be some flexibility in approach, depending on the needs of the situation as assessed at the time, and the response is purely the suggested, appropriate, logical solution.

Table 3.1 gives an indication as to a potential response, related directly to the level of threat perceived. Communication figures at all levels, as this must always be maintained, and no action should be taken without continued communication with clients, regardless of how aggressive they may seem. If clients are confused they will need to be reassured, even if physical techniques are being employed.

**Table 3.1** Common behaviour and suggested appropriate responses

| Client behaviour | Appropriate response |
|---|---|
| Compliant | Practitioner presence/communication |
| Verbal threat | Communications skills |
| Assaultive behaviour | Communication/breakaway techniques |
| Extreme violence | Communication/withdraw or intervention skills |

Physically intervening without assuring clients of what is happening will only serve to confuse and possibly anger them further. Continued communication gives clients an option to comply at any point in the proceedings but also gives provision for belated verbal de-escalation of the situation.

With respect to the responses cited, if clients were compliant, the mere presence of the practitioner would probably be enough to ensure that they moved back to their rooms or vacated the area, whichever was appropriate.

If verbal threats were being used service-providers should endeavour to use verbal communication skills to achieve agreement whereby both parties are satisfied and the conflict is resolved.

Assaultive behaviour includes low-intensity physical assaults, such as pushing, prodding or grabbing at clothing. These cannot be tolerated but it would be inappropriate and unethical to reply with either control skills or self-defence techniques such as strikes. Practitioners need either to leave the locale or to re-establish control, and consequently communication skills combined with non-aversive breakaway techniques would be recommended.

Extreme violence leaves practitioners liable to serious injury and therefore the primary consideration must be to withdraw to safety, accepting that the less time spent in the vicinity of the client, the less danger there is of coming to harm. If there is a duty of care to a client, or to others in the immediate area, it is reasonable to attempt an intervention or control skill, but only if there are enough people available to apply it effectively. Communication must not be forsaken in the haste to apply practical techniques.

Whereas the behaviour and responses are seemingly straightforward in principle, there is a third point on the conflict resolution plan that will have a large impression on the practicality and nature of the response elected; this is the 'impact factors'.

## IMPACT FACTORS

Impact factors are anything else that may have a bearing on the outcome of the situation and include issues such as the relative size, strength and age of the aggressor, any weapons they may be carrying or drugs they may have taken (prescribed or otherwise).

Common impact factors include the following.

## SIZE

The physical size of the client will determine what physical response may be appropriate. If the client is much bigger than the practitioner then certain breakaway or control techniques may prove ineffective. In the application of such techniques, reach and distance will be affected.

## AGE

If the client is elderly, and possibly infirm, it would be ill-advised to try an extreme controlling technique, primarily because of the potential for injury. Age may affect clients' ability to reason, and again, the practicality or effectiveness of a technique.

## SEX

It may prove inappropriate for a male practitioner to try and apply a control technique to a female client. A female practitioner may struggle to apply a breakaway or control technique to a larger male client. Similarly, a female client should not necessarily be left alone with male clients who may have any history of sexual irregularity. An attacker in a non-clinical confrontation may also be driven by a sexual motive.

## STRENGTH

If the client is physically much stronger than the practitioner, regardless of gender, again it may prove difficult to apply a breakaway or control technique effectively.

## ALCOHOL OR DRUGS

A significant impact factor is the effect of alcohol or drugs, either prescribed or otherwise. Already analysed as a causative factor, alcohol or drugs can make clients extremely difficult to handle, possibly lowering their inhibitions, increasing their confidence and distorting their perceptions.

## WEAPONS

If a client has a weapon, whether an actual recognized item, such as a knife, or merely something being employed as such, he or she immediately becomes harder to deal with, possibly dictating a greater degree of force being needed.

## NUMBER OF INDIVIDUALS

If there is more than one aggressor then the ability to manage the situation becomes increasingly difficult, particularly as other impact factors may well then be introduced, for example differing sizes, genders and strengths.

## FATIGUE

The aggressor may well be tired, limiting the ability to become involved in a protracted physical confrontation. Equally, the practitioner may be the tired party and feel unable, or actually be unable, to take control of the situation. This becomes more evident if the client has been exhibiting aggression and has spent excessive energies.

## INJURY

Either the client or practitioner may already be injured, possibly limiting their ability to function effectively or for a long duration.

## SKILL LEVEL

Practitioners with many years' experience in handling challenging behaviours may be more skilled and more confident to assume control. A new employee with relatively little experience and a low skill level could well feel unable to cope with a confrontation. Aggressors themselves may have some degree of high skill level, such as having previously served in the forces or studied some form of combat art.

## CLINICAL CONDITION

The client's actual condition may well prove a major impact factor (see causative factors, p. 14).

## VULNERABLE POSITION

Any location where the practitioner is in a disadvantaged position. If the aggressor is at the top of a flight of stairs while the practitioner is merely half-way up the same stairs, it may prove difficult to establish control from the position of vulnerability.

## KNOWLEDGE

Although not necessarily recognized as a core impact factor, it should also be considered that practitioners may have special knowledge of the clients' nature and of their condition that will affect their response. Practitioners must assess the potential threat in relation to this knowledge and consider the likelihood of clients becoming even more violent, or of resisting any attempts to reason or control.

## POTENTIAL IMPACT FACTORS – SUMMARY

- Size.
- Age.
- Strength.
- Gender.
- Numbers.
- Weapons.
- Vulnerable positioning.
- Alcohol or drugs.
- Clinical condition.
- Fatigue or injury.
- Skill level.
- Specialist knowledge.

## WARNING SIGNALS

Having already accepted that awareness is paramount in managing a situation and that it is vital to observe other people's body language, logically it must follow that the practitioner must know exactly what they are looking for. Clenched fists are a clear warning signal of a possible assault, but there are numerous other signs that are indicators that clients may be considering an attack, or may actually be at the point of doing so. These signals can be seen and measured to give advance warning of the individual's intention to attack.

When a threat is perceived, the body uses a biochemical system in order to prepare for 'fight or flight', through the release of adrenalin and noradrenalin. The nervous system utilizes two opposing systems: the 'go', which prepares the body for extreme activity; and the 'stop', which conserves energy and relaxes the body. Both these systems work as a counterbalance under normal conditions, but under provocation the body becomes primed for action and the 'go' assumes control.

If the client's facial colour darkens a physical attack is less likely owing to the 'go' system being undermined and the conflict being inhibited. Darkening in the face is a clear indicator that an individual is angry or frustrated, and certainly capable of aggression, but at that time the body is not actually prepared for the physical action itself. When the colour leaves the face and it lightens noticeably it is an indicator that the 'go' system is now taking control, transferring the blood from the skin and extremities to the muscle groups and vital organs where it will be needed.

Other warning signals include the following.

## BREATHING RATE

Accelerates as the body takes in more oxygen to prepare itself for extreme physical activity.

## ANIMATED MOVEMENTS

Large, animated movements indicate a surplus of adrenalin and emotion, both of which when combined in a frustrated person can lead to aggression.

## BOUNCING FROM FOOT TO FOOT

Using exaggerated foot movements indicates that an individual is working off a surplus of adrenalin and is therefore primed to launch a physical attack if the opportunity arises or if the frustration becomes too much to control.

## PROLONGED EYE CONTACT

Another warning signal, indicating the individual is working him- or herself up for a potential attack by fixating on the potential target.

## STANDING TALL

A common natural reaction as individuals try to make themselves look bigger and potentially more threatening, purely to intimidate their proposed target subject.

## CLENCHING AND UNCLENCHING OF FISTS

Also indicates the working off of excess adrenalin, only this time in a more obviously aggressive manner. The individual is using the adrenalin to prepare the body weapons to launch the assault.

## HANDS RISING ABOVE THE WAIST

Again, indicates that the individual is preparing to launch an assault. It is extremely difficult to launch a physical attack with the hands if they are below the waist.

## STANCE 'BLADES'

From 'straight on' into a sideways type stance, a natural defensive stance that provides some protection to the vital areas of the body, such as the groin, and a natural, subconscious reaction when humans prepare for combat.

## TARGET LOCATING

Occurs just prior to an attack when the individual will momentarily glance at the intended target, to make sure they connect with the assault.

## WARNING SIGNALS – SUMMARY

- Facial complexion darkens (reddens).
- Breathing accelerates.
- Animated hand gestures.
- Bouncing from foot to foot.
- Prolonged eye contact.
- Standing tall.
- Hands rising above waist.
- Stance 'blades'.
- Fists clench and unclench.
- Target locating.

Most warning signals will affect more traditional situations, such as Casualty departments or similar reception-orientated locations. In units dealing with severe mental health problems the clients are less likely to exhibit the traditionally recognized warning signals, depending very much on the nature of their individual conditions. However, some of the warning signals may still be exhibited and it is important that they are understood and that practitioners are fully aware so that they can identify them. The need to operate at condition 'yellow' becomes even more crucial if the signals are to be recognized.

Considering the three points on the conflict resolution plan, and then using the colour code to recognize early both a potential situation as well as any visible warning signals, will provide practitioners with all the information they need to formulate an appropriate, ethical response. The only factor not included within the equation is the practitioners' own belief systems, which will influence how they perceive the threat and therefore influence their actions.

Within traditional sociology a belief system may be defined as 'An imprint of more critical social myths and ideologies, knowledges and beliefs, whether they be drawn from the institutions of religion, magic, science, politics, or education as primary sources of ideas, or from secondary sources such as the media'.[18]

Everyone has their own belief system, but in a professional working environment, in particular a clinical situation where ethics and client care are paramount, these must not be allowed to impair the ability to take appropriate action. Whilst it is not normally possible to change an individual's belief system, and it should never really be attempted, it should not be contrary to the needs of the profession. Any perceived threat may be measured through an individual's belief system, and a response formulated on the basis of that belief system, but it must never transgress organizational policy for dealing with such episodes. The conflict resolution plan is an ideal principle to understand, it allows for a measured, appropriate and ethical response that can help to overcome any negative influences of an individual's belief system. In practice it is intended to provide a substitute belief system for application in the professional arena, although it may be applied to any situation.

Through a good sense of awareness of the environment and of all the individuals who will come into contact with it, provision may be made to deal with any aggressive incidents safely and ethically. The colour code may be used effectively to enhance self-awareness and a basic understanding of the conflict resolution plan, including the impact factors and warning signals, will often forewarn of an impending confrontation or assault. These are the basic elements that when combined will serve to greatly reduce the risk of a confrontation and, more importantly, will ensure that any such incident will be managed effectively.

# Chapter 4

# FEAR MANAGEMENT AND RESPONSES

## INTRODUCTION

It is a natural reaction for human beings to become nervous when under scrutiny or pressure. Athletes can often feel physically sick prior to an important event and for entertainers this can manifest itself as 'stage fright'. There are millions of people who are unable to stand up in front of an audience or a group of friends in order to give a speech, and yet for countless others it does not present any problem or fear whatsoever. Everybody is different and everybody responds differently to certain situations. When somebody is 'nervous' it is the body using its natural defence and releasing adrenalin.

Being 'nervous' is primarily a psychological condition induced by a fear of what may happen or go wrong, and the consequences of that failure, such as ridicule or loss of reward. The attack of 'nerves' can be so severe in some instances that the person concerned will feel physically nauseous or faint and may even pass out. Many people have a natural confidence and composure that allows them to maintain control and not succumb to this fear.

The 'nerves' experienced during a confrontation are brought on by a very real fear of coming to harm and are amplified. Very few people will be spared from feeling nervous during a physical confrontation and everybody will experience some form of physical and psychological change under such a situation.

## FIGHT OR FLIGHT?

When involved in any confrontation, whether verbal or physical, the body utilizes a biochemical system to prepare it for appropriate action. When threatened the body automatically releases adrenalin and noradrenalin as the individual prepares either to retaliate or to withdraw. This is often termed 'fight or flight'.

Adrenalin is a hormone that is released into the body during stress situations and is essential to survival in a threatening situation, where a physical encounter is unavoidable. Both attackers and defenders will utilize adrenalin, although possibly in different ways. The hormone allows the body to achieve its maximum potential but is generally released in a burst or 'adrenalin dump'.

'Fight of flight' refers to the adrenalin dump being used in different ways. Some people will use the adrenalin to maximize the physical attack, others will use it to maximize their running ability in order to escape.

The human body prepares itself for action using the nervous system. As mentioned earlier (see Chapter 3) this comprises two opposing systems: the 'go' system prepares the body for action; and the 'stop' system gives signals to relax and conserve energy. Under normal conditions the body responds to both systems and an even balance is maintained. When under threat or pressure, the 'stop' system will be overridden and the body prepared for action.

## IN A CONFRONTATION

When involved in a confrontation it is reasonable to measure the threat faced by assessing an opponent's behaviour. White-faced, tight-lipped individuals are very capable of launching a physical assault as the body has prepared them for action by transferring blood from the skin in order to protect the vital organs. Carbohydrate floods the blood with sugar in order to provide maximum energy and their breathing becomes quicker and deeper, preparing them for combat. Red-faced individuals, however, are less likely to attack as the conflict is being inhibited and undermined by the 'stop' system.

In a defence situation, when adrenalin is released the heart rate also increases. When the heart rate reaches approximately 115 beats per minute, fine motor skills such as restraint techniques will begin to fail. When the heart rate exceeds around 145 beats per minute the visual system begins to narrow and complex motor skills, which involve co-ordination and timing, will deteriorate. For individuals who are hoping to control or contain a violent encounter the increasing heartbeat will seriously affect their ability to do so. The less confident a person is the higher the heart rate will increase and the more adrenalin will be released. At this level if no response is initiated individuals will begin to feel a degree of confusion and may also experience nausea.

When the heart rate exceeds around 175 beats per minute, individuals will suffer loss of peripheral vision (tunnel vision), along with auditory exclusion. Depth of perception will also fail and they will see objects as closer or further away than they actually are. At this level there is often a complete failure of cognitive abilities, which can result in freezing or wild irrational acts, such as lunging for an opponent. At this level, if no physical action is undertaken the body may simply just shut down, resulting in individuals passing out. The examples are based upon an average healthy adult with a resting heart rate of between 60 and 80 beats per minute. Whilst different individuals will have varying resting heart rates, the benchmark intervals remain proportionately constant with respect to physical and psychological change or impediment under pressure.

Techniques relying on gross motor skills improve as the heart rate increases, but as reasoning fails at a proportionate rate they will often be delivered blindly. Combat sports and martial arts rely heavily on gross motor skill techniques, such as kicks and punches, which is why they are often extremely effective under pressure, even after a low level of training. The problem is that the use of techniques from such systems without any cognitive control may well be futile, or, alternatively, could prove fatal. Certainly, it is not recommended to rely on such moves in a working environment.

In simple terms, when under threat, individuals will resort to gross motor skills – basic techniques that they know will work. When the 'go' system takes control there will automatically be physical and psychological changes occurring within the body, such as a raised heart rate, which in turn will help to accelerate respiration and increase the levels of adrenalin. Unless individuals elect to withdraw from the situation they must be prepared either to fight, using gross motor skills, or to regain control of their body and manage their fear.

In order to regain control of the body it is important to slow down the heart rate and free off the secondary nervous system that controls the body's natural defence mechanism. This is located in the centre of the torso at the solar plexus. The easiest way to regain control is to slow down the respiration by breathing deeply and slowly, so expanding the chest and freeing off tension at the solar plexus. This, in turn, will slow down the heart rate and allow blood to circulate more naturally and the mind to function more clearly. Breathing in this way will not occur automatically, hence a deliberate and concentrated effort must be made by individuals to do so. Once this has been instigated, control and the ability to reason can resume fairly quickly, but it is important not to make the breathing too apparent as a potential adversary may identify it as weakness and an opportune moment to launch an attack.

In addition to the 'fight or flight' response there is also a third common reaction when individuals come under attack. Quite often individuals cannot comprehend what is happening to them, or why it is happening, and they simply freeze, consequently becoming unable to escape or to formulate any form of defence. This occurs due to a complete failure of cognitive abilities, resulting from either the surprise of the attack or a lack of experience, training or understanding of aggression, awareness or of defence strategies. There will still be a release of adrenalin or noradrenalin but whilst under pressure and not understanding the attack, the body cannot determine whether to 'go' or 'stop' and as a result no action is taken.

## WHY STUDY AGGRESSION MANAGEMENT TECHNIQUES?

Studying aggression management, combined with a grounding in basic defence techniques, will, in the majority of instances, preclude an individual from freezing when under threat. Merely understanding that anybody can become subject to an assault and that there are appropriate measures to take under such instances can make a significant difference to individuals' responses. Freezing is a non-reaction, induced primarily because victims have no defence strategy to draw upon and cannot control the body.

Merely understanding the principles of violence and aggression enables individuals to identify potential problems in advance and equips them with the skills necessary to manage the situation effectively. In short, it will give them a strategy, whereas before there would have been none, even if that strategy is simply to employ deep breathing to try and regain control.

Being completely aware of self and surroundings is vital to promoting effective personal safety and the positive management of any aggressive situation. By identifying potential problems early the body can begin to prepare itself and strategies for escape or defence may be explored. At the point of recognizing a threat, deep-breathing techniques may be employed to ensure that control is maintained for as long as is necessary. Knowing that control can be maintained and that defence is possible can increase both confidence and effectiveness.

Experience, training and knowledge are all factors that instil confidence and self-belief. When individuals believe that they can succeed they have a good chance of doing so. If, on the other hand, they do not believe they can achieve something, they will rarely rise to the challenge of actually doing so. Similarly, believing in the ability to control or protect oneself is the first step towards being able to do so. If someone does not believe that their strategy or technique will work, there is no point in them trying it because it will not!

Chapter 5

# VERBAL CONFRONTATIONS AND COMMUNICATION

## INTRODUCTION

Severe or persistent verbal abuse can cause considerable distress to victims, which could result in anxiety or stress, affecting their health and ability to work. Should verbal abuse be allowed to continue unchecked, either from clients or co-workers, it can easily progress into a physical assault. Many physical assaults are preceded by some form of verbal exchange. If a situation is handled correctly at the verbal stage then it is possible to diffuse it completely.

Should individuals be physically assaulted, with no warning or preceding verbal interaction, the only response open to them would be the use of practical techniques. Whilst defending themselves it may be possible, although unlikely, to reason with an aggressor in order to stop the attack. This can prove extremely difficult, particularly if an assailant has gained an advantage. However, had there been some initial dialogue, victims may have been able to prevent the situation escalating into violence.

Aggressors who are intent on physically attacking someone will possibly do so without any prior warning, enabling them to gain the upper hand. Someone who initially threatens or questions their intended target may not be entirely confident of either their motivating facts, or of their ability to win. If they gain satisfaction within a verbal exchange they can avoid a physical confrontation that they themselves sometimes do not even want.

In a working situation it is possible for people to become agitated or frustrated if they cannot get their own way. Abusive clients and heated negotiations or interviews can seriously affect service-providers' health and if handled badly can lead to physical assaults. Some individuals can be very assertive and manipulative, which can also result in the service-providers themselves becoming resentful or angry.

A verbal exchange indicates a problem that needs resolving and the first and most important thing to do is concentrate on that *problem*, and not the other person, no matter how difficult or aggressive he or she may be. The problem has to be understood fully and therefore it is vital to listen. Should service-providers not understand the problem or, worse still, not know that there is one, they will not be able to resolve it. Communication needs to be encouraged rather than ended.

## COMMUNICATION

If an assault begins verbally it is an opportunity, albeit difficult, to communicate. The other person must be encouraged to talk. Listening is an excellent method of calming a situation. Aggressors may well want to explain their concerns and listening allows them to do so. It is common for complainants to show an initial burst of anger as a result of adrenalin and anxiety but this will soon subside if they are handled correctly. In any situation anger must not be met with anger, as this will only escalate hostilities and destroy the communication process.

It is not easy to remain calm when under threat or pressure, but attempting to do so will help the situation and can lead to a calming of both parties. Service-providers must not only listen, but must be seen to be listening. Individuals with problems require undivided attention, particularly if they are also angry. Simple gestures, such as a nod or verbal acknowledgment, show clearly that attention is being paid.

If practicable, aggressors should be offered a seat at the earliest opportunity. This is a personal gesture that will help to assure them that their issue is being taken seriously and that there is no desire merely to remove them quickly from the establishment. Sitting down is automatically more relaxing and therefore will assist in the calming process. More importantly, it puts both aggressors and service-providers at the same level, taking away any physical or psychological advantage that may be gained by having one person standing over the other, especially if there is a significant difference in physical size. Lastly, it should be considered that it is harder to launch a physical assault from a seated position, and if an attempt is made, it is seen more easily.

Hospitality can be a very positive defensive tool. Offering a seat, or even a drink, is a recognized gesture of consideration and may instantly diffuse an aggressive situation and commence the communication process. However, should aggressors refuse to be seated then both parties should remain standing, but with consideration to the distance between them.

Regardless of the nature of the issue concerned, neither side should be judgemental, although aggressors will probably already have firmly established their own perceptions. All words used need to be selected carefully and delivered calmly and openly, avoiding emotion. With a significant amount of communication being translated through body language and not words, this must compliment what is actually being said. When listening, body language needs to illustrate genuine interest or concern.

With respect to feelings and attitudes, only approximately seven per cent are communicated with actual words. Approximately 38 per cent of the message is received through the tone of the voice and, more importantly, as much as 55 per cent is conveyed through body language. With this in mind it is even more important to monitor our own personal feelings with regard to the issue being discussed, and ensure these are not conveyed to the other person unless intended.

## COMMUNICATION – SUMMARY

Feelings and attitudes are communicated:

- Approximately seven per cent through the actual *words* used.
- Approximately 38 per cent through the *tone* of the voice.
- Approximately 55 per cent through *body language*.

'Checking' is a useful technique to help the communication process, to calm complainants and, more significantly, to ensure that all the facts are understood. This process involves restating any key information that has been divulged, therefore showing aggressors that the other party is actually listening to them and has a correct understanding of the problem. It is vital when checking to let aggressors say everything they need to say before attempting to resolve any issue. Interrupting them will stop the flow of information, some of which may be vital, and may also anger them further.

Even as complainants explain their problems they may well still show signs of anger or frustration, but once they have actually stated their point, there is an opportunity to use the checking techniques. A positive response at this stage would be, *'Now, I would just like to make sure I've got everything right. You say that you want* (or need) . . .', etc. Once stated, the subject matter may be reaffirmed, *'Is that correct? Is there anything else I can do for you?'*

The closing question will ensure that the whole issue has been divulged and that all problems are presented. An open question such as this may invite a further outburst of aggression but it demonstrates clearly that service-providers are listening and aim to help, whilst ensuring all the relevant information is obtained.

Checking in this manner shows immediately that service-providers have been paying attention and that they are interested enough to ensure that they get the facts right. This will instill confidence that the matter will be attended to. It is often good practice when checking to take notes of the key points, although always ask permission to do so first, using a simple request such as, *'Do you mind if I take notes to make sure I don't miss anything?'*

Note-taking will ensure that nothing is missed and that the facts of the issue are recorded correctly. Simply suggesting that notes be taken can help to calm complainants and reassure them that action will be taken. Merely requesting to do so shows consideration and intent to take the matter seriously. The notes can be referred to in the checking process. Checking also allows service-providers to show comprehension of the issues concerned and to confirm visibly that understanding. Despite the validity of taking notes, always remember that if complainants are highly abusive or very aggressive it would not be advisable to do so without first requesting permission.

Once all the information has been checked, and complainants have acknowledged this, an attempt can be made to resolve the issue. If service-providers are not in a position to offer a solution, or do not have the necessary knowledge to do so, they should go and seek assistance. It is vital to be honest and keep complainants informed. A simple 'withdrawal statement' would be, *'I'm sorry but I'm not able to resolve this but now I have all the facts I will go and get somebody who can help you. If you'd just like to wait here I won't be very long.'* This statement is simple, concise and yet honest and positive.

During the checking process it is possible that complainants may still exhibit aggressive behaviour. Checking requires communication from both sides and it may prove easier at this time to reason with them more directly. Once an intention to assist has been established it can be readily reinforced with a simple disarming statement, *'I'm here to help you solve this but I can't unless you stop shouting at me!'*

If complainants continue to be abusive and threatening, without any signs of calming, then it may be necessary to withdraw before or during the checking process. A similar withdrawal statement can also be used, but in this instance it is not necessarily to resolve a problem, but to gain assistance and to ensure personal safety. Anybody who feels they are in physical danger should always withdraw and seek assistance.

## OPEN AND CLOSED QUESTIONS

More information may be required to help calm a situation or resolve a problem. Asking relevant questions will also demonstrate a willingness to resolve differences. The use of specific 'open' questions will ensure the correct information is obtained. An example would be, *'When exactly did the problem start?'* This question requires useful information to be exchanged in return, promoting further verbal communication. A 'closed' question would be, *'Has this been going on for long?'*, which could be answered with a simple 'yes' or 'no'. Although the two example questions may sound similar, the latter will restrict communication and encourage more simplistic, possibly abrupt answers.

If somebody is physically injured they may be in pain and as a result demonstrate uncharacteristic aggression. In this instance appropriate treatment will help to manage the situation but the logical approach for communication would be to ask, *'Where exactly does it hurt?'*, as opposed to, *'Does it hurt?'*

There are six basic open questions that require information to be exchanged: 'Who?', 'When?', 'Where?', 'Why?', 'What?' and 'How?'. It may also be prudent to ask a 'high gain' question in order to obtain more comprehensive information and to make complainants think more carefully about the answer. An appropriate high gain question may be, *'What is the one thing I could do for you that would really help your situation?'* This type of question generally requires complainants to consider their answer and to use some reasoning. Once they start reasoning they are less likely to become aggressive because they are using cognitive abilities as opposed to being controlled by their emotions.

## OPEN QUESTIONS

To be used to gain productive information:

- Who?
- When?
- Where?
- Why?
- What?
- How?

Questions need to be used carefully and selected with tact. If it is not obvious why the question is being asked then the reason for using it should be stated, *'In order for me to treat you I need to know exactly when the problem began?'* A question of this nature tells complainants what information is required and why it is needed. Even in a delicate situation personal questions can be asked, provided they are justified and tact is used.

It is recommended that service-providers appear positive, even if it is not possible to agree with complainants' problems or points of view. It is possible to instill confidence by use of a positive statement, whilst not actually agreeing with the other party or admitting any responsibility or fault, *'I can see what you're saying to me now!'* or, *'I understand your point of view!'* are both very positive-sounding statements, but neither are actually saying that the complainant is right or that the service-provider is wrong.

## THE OTHER PERSPECTIVE

When attempting to resolve an issue it is very important to try and see the other person's perspective. Acknowledging other people and their problems is the first step towards resolving the matter. If dealing with personal issues, practitioners should be empathetic, but never sympathetic, as this can be perceived as patronizing but also may lead to personal or emotional involvement beyond a professional capacity.

The use of 'personal disclosure' may also be relevant and could help complainants to rationalize their problems and not feel that they are on their own. A personal disclosure entails listeners relaying a similar relevant experience that they have had or been involved with, illustrating that they can relate to the matter at hand. The use of such a tactic, however, must be considered carefully as it is encouraging a more personal response, potentially weakening a professional relationship, which may prove difficult to re-establish later.

Although certain situations may require some form of disclosure it is better, where possible, to concentrate solely on the facts, particularly if complainants are very aggressive in their attitude. Being direct and straightforward will avoid getting sidetracked into irrelevent issues. Only the truth must be offered and if it is necessary to return any information it is good practice, if practicable, to use some form of illustration. This can help to ensure a clear understanding and a lack of any confusion. Complex terms should also be avoided if at all possible.

In some instances individuals will not accept any information that is given to them. If the information is key to resolving their problem, or to calming the situation, it needs to be relayed as many times as is necessary for them to understand and accept. This will require the use of the 'broken record' principle.

A continuous, clear repetition of the relevant information or feelings will often be required to stop people from criticizing or pressuring. It need not be exactly the same sentence or phrase that is used, provided the message remains constant. Complainants may try and distract service-providers by raising other issues. They are merely trying to avoid the message and therefore it must be continued until it is acknowledged. Once accepted any other issues may be addressed as necessary. But by sticking to the point complainants will eventually realize that they are only ever going to get one answer.

Humour should only ever be used with caution. It can be used effectively to take the heat from a potentially volatile situation, but should be employed selectively. Any humour used should not denegrate complainants or their problems. Similarly, it should not be detrimental to individuals using it or the organization they represent, which would open further the gap between service-providers and clients.

Certain issues cannot be resolved at the time of the confrontation, although there will nearly always be pressure for an immediate response. If an issue cannot be resolved or is in danger of escalating then it becomes vital to gain more time to think. It is reasonable to ask for time to consider a response. Having listened and checked, it is advisable to use a 'withdrawal statement' such as, *'I understand your problem, but I need time to check some information before I can resolve it. I can let you know later.'*

If a problem cannot be resolved at that moment, it is good practice to give a projected time for the matter to be settled. This should be realistic and adhered to. If there is an extended period envisaged, complainants should be updated periodically as to the status of their issue. Similarly, they should be notified if there is to be any delay, including the reasons for it.

## KEEP PEOPLE INFORMED

One of the biggest catalysts of violent and aggressive behaviour is people not being kept informed about a matter that they feel is important. As a part of their job service-providers will not always see others' problems as being overly important, particularly if they are dealing with a large number of cases at the same time. To the individual concerned, however, the case may be of the utmost importance and urgency.

Some people may have a number of problems that need resolving, even though their anger may be focused into one particular issue. Once all the information has been received and checked it can be an effective tactic to direct complainants to one of the issues that may be resolved more easily. By doing this individuals can see that some progress is being made.

After all the questioning and all the attempts to calm complainants it may still be necessary to say, 'No'. This can often trigger further violence and aggression. There are many ways to refuse a request but in order to avoid confusion it is necessary to say, 'No' as early as possible, and then stick to it. The message needs to be delivered politely and it should be recognized that the refusal may cause difficulties or even resentment. The reasons for a refusal can be stated in order to diffuse a difficult situation, but they are never to be considered as open for discussion as this may encourage complainants to believe the decision is reversible, or may just simply anger them further. Service-providers are there to assist and subsequently should help complainants to focus on any alternatives or possibilities beyond the refusal.

Obviously, not all verbal confrontations occur in the workplace, but the principles employed to handle any incident are basically the same. If aggressors intend to assault somebody in the street they normally do so without any prior verbal exchange. If they confront verbally first, it is likely that they are either unsure of their ability to win or are unsure of their justification for the confrontation.

Examples of commonly used opening lines are, '*What are you looking at?*' or, '*What have you been saying about me?*' Both these statements are extremely confrontational and are used specifically to measure a reaction. Aggressors are waiting to see how confident their target is, or is making sure that their motives are correct. If victims show weakness it fuels aggressors' confidence and they will feel in a stronger position to progress the confrontation. Similarly, if victims confirm the motive, or apologize for the suggested transgression, aggressors will feel justified in their subsequent course of action.

The opening line is an invitation to commence the communication process. Defenders must remain calm and in control, measuring their responses and choosing their words carefully. The further the conversation progresses, the less likely aggressors are to assault physically. If the opening line had been, *'What have you been saying about me?'*, a questioning approach may be employed to further the verbal communication. *'Nothing. Why? What have you heard?'* is a possible response, inviting more information to be returned, checked and then confidently and politely dismissed. Placing doubt in the attacker's mind is the logical way to diffuse a situation. If the response was, *'I said you were incompetent, and you are!'*, the situation will escalate rapidly.

In the instance of a statement such as, *'What are you looking at?'*, an appropriate response might be a confident, *'I'm sorry, I didn't realize I was looking.'* This return statement, if delivered politely and with confidence, whilst showing no weakness or aggression, will help to eliminate aggressors' reasons for pursuing an attack.

In any response situation the body language must correspond with what is actually being said. Not forgetting that the majority of messages communicated are through gestures rather than by the actual words being spoken is equally important. If the gestures contradict what is being said aggressors are likely to get the wrong message, which can serve to fuel further the confrontation.

## BODY LANGUAGE

The following examples illustrate commonly encountered body language. Although they are acknowledged as being excellent indicators, they should never be accepted as truly definitive. Clever or manipulative individuals will deliberately mislead through controlling or directing their body language. With experience this can sometimes be identified, as it is often difficult to control or sustain 'fake' body language for an extended period. It would be prudent to treat all individuals with caution until a proper assessment can be made. The illustrations can also be used by the reader to identify and measure their own body language.

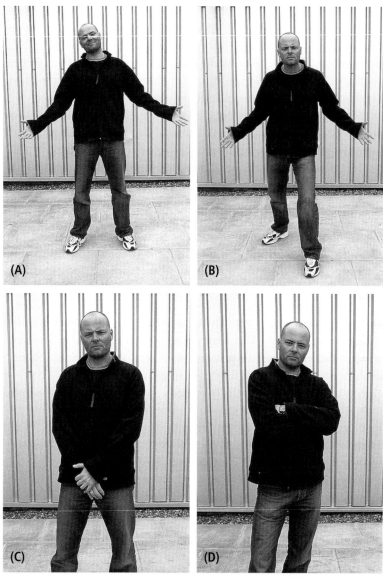

**Figure 5.1** (A) Openness gesture. Fully exposed palms, head in neutral position, communicating a non-threatening attitude. Facial expression reinforces gestures. (B) Openly aggressive. Although the body position is similar to (A), this is giving aggressive signals due to the upper body leaning forward and the stern facial expression. (C) Partial arm barrier covering the groin. Defensive stance, indicating a possible lack of confidence. (D) Basic arm barrier. Negative in gesture, the crossed arms may conceal a potential weapon.

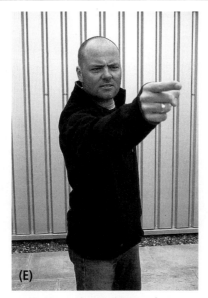

**Figure 5.1** (E) Direct pointing, a clear indicator of aggression.

## A PROFESSIONAL APPROACH

When considering body language it should be remembered that feelings and attitudes are readily communicated in this way. Although words may convey data, facts and information, it is the body language which communicates attitudes, feelings and emotions, including possibly even intent.

The following are to be considered.

## POSTURE

Standing straight with head held high indicates assertiveness. If the chin is down and the head ducked this indicates potential vulnerability. Shoulders should always be relaxed and hands open. Fists should never be clenched and pointing finger gestures are to be totally avoided. Clients who drop the chin may also indicate that they are about to attack, especially if they have adopted a 'bladed' stance and raised their hands above the waist. In this instance, dropping the head is a reflex action to protect the throat whilst in combat.

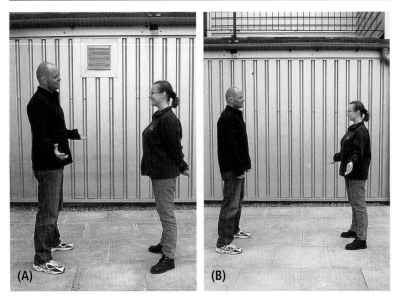

**Figure 5.2** (A) Both parties willing to communicate, that is, both relaxed, subject with open gestures, possibly to encourage communication. Practitioner (on right) has hands behind her back – non-threatening but leaving her potentially vulnerable. (B) Practitioner (on right) maintaining a good reactionary gap and using open hand gestures to enhance communication, whilst keeping the hands free to use as a barrier between her and the agressor, should the need arise.

## DISTANCE

A comfortable relaxed distance needs to be maintained. Stand too close to a person and they may feel as though their personal space has been invaded. Too far away and they will feel distant and removed. For defensive purposes practitioners should try and maintain a 'reactionary gap' of between two and four metres. Closer than this makes defence very difficult, if not impossible.

## EYES

Fear or aggression can often be seen in a person's eyes. An old saying is that, 'The eyes are the windows of the soul'. To some extent this may be true. Eye contact should be maintained at all times, as this is seen as being approachable and indicates honesty and integrity, provided it is supported by an appropriate facial expression, such as smiling. Staring, however, often has the opposite effect, indicating intensity or potential hostility. Avoiding eye contact or wearing dark glasses can be perceived as lacking in confidence or hiding something.

## MOUTH AND JAW

Facial expressions must match body gestures and the words being spoken. A false smile can be readily identified as just that. A genuine smile will prove a positive method of reassuring and relaxing other people.

## VOICE

Always speak slowly and clearly to ensure that everything is understood. Speaking too loudly or too softly may prove either irritating or intimidating. Speaking quickly is an indicator of not being in control – either through being nervous and unconfident – or through being overly confident and not taking the time to consider what is being said. In order to maintain interest it is good practice to vary the pitch and the tone of the voice.

## GESTURES

Body language cover most aspects of body or hand gestures, but it is simple to remember that folded arms indicate a defensive or non-commital stance and may also conceal a potential weapon. Hands on hips or pointing fingers are indicators of aggression. Fiddling gestures, or constant nervous movements, such as rubbing the hands together, can be very irritating but may also be perceived as a lack of confidence or having something to hide. Raising the hands above the waist may indicate that an aggressor is preparing to launch an attack, particularly if a 'side on' stance has been adopted.

## APPEARANCE

Clothing and choice of hairstyle indicates personal style or character. It is always beneficial to establish a personal style that is appropriate for the mood of the situation. Dressing inappropriately may give confusing signals and prompt a confrontation, based purely upon appearance. Similarly, an extreme physical appearance may prompt assumptions from others and fuel certain prejudices, which in turn may be used as ammunition during a verbal exchange, or as a motive for a physical attack.

From a risk management perspective it is always prudent to wear clothes appropriate to the task and of no high fiscal or sentimental value. Working in high-heeled shoes or tight skirts may prove impractical, but trying to execute any defensive techniques may prove almost impossible in such attire. If working with a client known to be violent it should be taken for granted that clothes could be ripped or stained.

One of the most commonly used hand gestures in Western society is to shake hands as a greeting or farewell. If a person shakes hands with the palm face down then they are generally seen as taking control of the situation. Shaking hands with the palm face up is perceived as giving control. A logical non-confrontational compromise is to give the hand in a straight position with the palm sideways. Using a firm grip whilst shaking hands is a sign of assertiveness and confidence. A weak handshake can be perceived as being timid or weak, but equally, too strong a grip may be seen as aggressive or an attempt to dominate.

As with any body language, individuals may deliberately mislead by their dress, voice or any other gesture. In order to get what they want some individuals learn how to control their body language and their gestures. They consider carefully what clothes they should wear and how they should pitch their voice in order to manipulate other people. All aspects of their presentation build up into a complete picture and consequently it is important to assess each factor of their persona. It is not uncommon for an aggressive individual to deliberately act friendly in order to relax the potential victim and keep them off guard.

## APPEARING CONFIDENT

Having looked at different types of body language, and assertained how important it is to project the right image, the following are useful pointers to ensure that service-providers appear confident and capable. To achieve this the following attitudes should be applied:

- Always approach people directly and smile.
- Always look into the other person's face or eyes (but avoid staring).
- Always keep the head held up.
- If appropriate, shake hands firmly and confidently.
- When talking keep the hands away from the face.
- If standing, use only open hand gestures or, if not confident enough, keep hands still by the sides of the body.

- If seated, sit back into the chair and relax. Avoid perching on the front of the seat.
- Stay relatively still, using slow movements. Avoid wriggling or any large, animated movements.
- Endeavour to relax and speak slowly and clearly.
- If an error is made, acknowledge it and move on. Do not try to hide it.

## COMMUNICATION INFORMATION

In any situation where verbal interaction is used, whether at work, or socially, only a limited amount of what is said will ever actually be understood. In a formal interview situation there is a possibility that slightly more information may be retained, but Table 5.1 provides an approximation of the effectiveness of communicating specific information.

The information in Table 5.1 obviously reinforces the need to speak slowly and clearly and to keep all information as simple as possible. If possible, visual aids and supportive written information should be used to enhance receivers' ability to understand and retain the message that is being given to them. The approximate percentage of information that can be retained under different circumstances is shown in Table 5.2.

The statistics shown in Table 5.2 are based purely on a limited time span immediately after a meeting or interview. Obviously, with the passage of time retention of information drops considerably and the more time that passes, the more will be forgotten. But the impor-

**Table 5.1** Communicating information

| Information communicated | Percentage efficiency of communication |
|---|---|
| What we actually want to say | 100 |
| What we actually say | 80 |
| What is understood by the other person | 60 |
| What is accepted by the other person | 30 |
| What is retained by the other person | 20 |

**Table 5.2** Information retention

| Information source | Percentage retained |
| --- | --- |
| What is read | 10 |
| What is heard | 20 |
| What is seen | 30 |
| What is seen and heard | 50 |
| What is said | 70 |
| What is said and done | 90 |

tant factor to remember is that in order to manage an awkward interview or a difficult verbal confrontation successfully it is paramount that the listener understands the message that is being transmitted. Confusion leads to frustration and, in extreme instances, aggression.

In a working environment it is often possible to take control of a situation or to set the tone of a meeting or interview by carefully considering the layout of the room. How much information is gained from an interview, or how relaxed a session is, may be controlled to a certain extent.

## POSITIVE COMMUNICATION

Service-providers may have an understanding of body language, and may have taken the time to consider the layout of a proposed interview room, but further consideration must also be given to what is actually going to be communicated. A definition of communication is 'the transmission of an idea or message so that the sender and the receiver have the same understanding'.

It is important that this is accepted from the outset, otherwise any attempted communication could break down. There are a number of reasons why communication fails.

- Service-providers assume too much of clients, instead of ascertaining and then 'checking' the facts. It is common for service-providers merely to forge ahead. This makes clients feel isolated and fails to achieve the 'same understanding'.

- Service-providers are ambiguous, unintentionally or deliberately, failing to make important points clear, or attempting to confuse on purpose.
- Service-providers do not listen to other people and fail to consult them.
- Service-providers are too technical or too complicated in their terminology.
- Too much control is taken of the situation, not allowing clients to participate.
- Not enough facts or knowledge are used to get the message across clearly.
- A failure to speak the 'same language' as the receiver, that is, to estrange the other person through the use of certain terms, diction, phrases or dialect.

All the above may cause a breakdown in communication. For an interview to be both relaxed and successful, good communicators must ask open questions in order to gain relevant information and to encourage communication, listen to the answers and endeavour to speak the same language.

To enhance communication:

- Ask open questions.
- Listen to the answers.
- Speak the same language.

Further to this, interviewers must also consider what they actually wish to achieve and, therefore, what they wish to say themselves and why. When considering the approach to be taken, and the questions to be asked, thought should be given to what reaction will be encountered. Do clients have enough knowledge of the issue to be able to understand the situation, or will they need additional support or information?

There are other barriers to communication that can prompt frustration and possibly lead to increased tension. The following are the most common ones.

Lack of enough time to cover the subject and resolve the issue. Enough time must be allocated to deal properly with any problem. If time is not available then an attempt should be made to resolve part of the issue or to give the other person positive information that the matter will be satisfactorily dealt with, and when this will be done (see also p. 50).

Clients will sometimes not allow communication. In this situation it is a good strategy to let them talk themselves out and merely listen. Whilst clients are talking they are imparting potentially valuable information that could subsequently be of use, but more importantly they are not using physical aggression.

It is also possible for clients to think they have more knowledge than service-providers. This is a difficult scenario to manage but these clients must be encouraged to air their opinions or ideas, and then an attempt made to tactfully correct them if it is necessary or productive to do so. Often, clients will only hear what they want to hear and therefore supportive evidence, such as documentation, may serve to make the process easier. Service-providers may need to use the 'broken record' strategy (see p. 49) to ensure the correct message is finally acknowledged.

Interruptions can be extremely damaging to an interview if progress is being made. A potentially aggressive client will command undivided attention and this should be given. Service-providers should never allow themselves to be drawn away from the matter in hand, other than deliberately for safety reasons, or to be distracted into other conversations or tasks.

So, barriers to communication include:

- Lack of time allocated to resolve the issue.
- Negative or domineering attitude of either person.
- Preconceived ideas contrary to the facts.
- Interruptions.

There are several aids to communication that can ensure the message is understood by the interviewee, as follows.

Practitioners should have a complete knowledge of the subject. If not, then the issue needs to be referred to somebody who has the appropriate knowledge, or, ideally, it should be researched before the interview. Research may mean that the interview would need to be rescheduled, but it is strategically better than holding a meeting that cannot be concluded satisfactorily through ignorance of the facts. Providing inaccurate information will only create further problems and an increased sense of frustration.

Interviewers must establish feedback from clients.

The matter should be simplified in order to avoid confusion and ensure that the message is received clearly. Overcomplication results in frustration, confusion and alienation, which with an already anxious subject may result in a serious threat of violence.

The use of visual aids or demonstrations reinforces understanding and will also make it easier to explain the facts.

Aids to communication include:

- Knowledge.
- Establishing feedback.
- Keeping the matter as simple as possible.
- Visual aids and demonstrations.

## INTERVIEWS

There are a number of interviewing scenarios that need to be treated with tact and consideration in order to ensure a positive outcome is achieved. Disciplinary or appraisal interviews will often place subordinates under close scrutiny and they can become either defensive or aggressive.

Managers need to have all the facts before the interview. In a disciplinary situation there will normally be a specific problem area, which may be identified as a 'gap' between the expectations of the establishment and the compliance of subordinates. In any interaction situation where there is a problem or disagreement this could also be termed as a 'gap'.

A logical procedure to manage such an interview effectively is as follows:

Establish the *gap*. First, both parties must identify and agree exactly what the problem is.

Focus on the *facts*. Only the facts need to be considered. Nothing else is relevant. Subordinates need to be given an opportunity to speak for themselves, and hence should be encouraged to talk. This will probably gain all the information required about how the situation arose and what subordinates expect to be done about it, by both the establishment and themselves. Open questions should be used to ensure all the key facts are presented. Managers must then listen and acknowledge those facts.

*Agree* on the area of the gap. Having explored the gap by asking questions and listening, both parties must now agree on what exactly the problem is.

*Eliminate* the gap. Once agreement has been reached, an appropriate course of action may be decided. Set targets for subordinates to aim for in respect of them meeting the expectations of the organization. This may be a time-based target, for subordinates to resolve their concerns or improve their performance. It could also be a productivity target. Any target set must be achievable, realistic and agreed by both parties.

Fix a *review* date. In order to measure the success of the meeting, a further review interview should be arranged. This allows an opportunity to assess whether the 'gap' has been closed or whether any additional issues need resolving. If a target has been set then the review is the logical time to appraise the performance against the goal.

It is professional practice in disciplinary interviews, in particular those relating to serious matters of misconduct, for subordinates to be allowed an independent witness, or in extreme instances even some form of legal representation. Management, too, should not be solely represented by one individual in these instances. Taking notes and recording all facts becomes increasingly important in this situation.

Minor infringements or poor performance issues may be managed by use of the above method, possibly at appraisal time, without necessarily involving third parties, although this is still an option.

The steps of the interview listed above should be followed closely in order to achieve a positive outcome. It is common for managers to try and sell their solution before wholly understanding the full extent of the problem. This merely creates frustration in subordinates, which can then manifest itself in aggression. Managers need to guide the interview to some extent, but they must be prepared to share the talking and listen to exactly what subordinates are saying. There will occasionally be pauses in responses which need to be respected in order for subordinates to formulate the answers they want. Hard prompting during pauses will also create frustration and resentment.

If the issue under discussion is complex, it is good to summarize periodically. Criticism only ever has a negative effect on individuals, and should never be introduced into any interview or meeting. If managers or the establishment have areas that need improving, or that may have been at fault, these too need to be acknowledged, but no liability for the actual core problem should be accepted without careful consideration and consultation, probably through more senior management. No promises should ever be made that cannot be kept.

At the end of any appraisal, no matter how bad, or any disciplinary meeting, it is important to close with some positive statements. Subordinates will probably feel relieved that the problem has been addressed but could also feel low or depressed. Ending on a positive note will help their self-esteem, but will also reassure them that there is an end to the matter in sight.

A poorly handled appraisal or disciplinary interview can lead to resentment, frustration, anger and even physical aggression. Responsible managers know their people well and will be watching for any signs of an existing or potential problem. Once managers have identified a problem they should then arrange a counselling interview.

## INTERVIEWING DIFFICULT INTERVIEWEES

All people are different, with differing principles and belief systems, but there are certain individuals who can prove particularly awkward in an interview situation. The following can present themselves during an interview.

'The Buck Passer', who is never to blame. It is always someone or something else that was responsible. In this instance managers need to be 100 per cent convinced of their facts and have all relevant information available.

'The Injured Innocent', who always assumes an innocent and injured perspective, using statements such as, *'Surely, you don't think I would do such a thing deliberately?'* Again, managers must be totally convinced of their facts and have all relevant evidence readily to hand.

'The Counter Attacker', whose philosophy is, 'the best form of defence is attack!'. This person will try and turn the interview around into an attack on managers, the organization or their colleagues. Whilst it is generally a verbal onslaught, such as, *'Alright, let's have it out, right now!'* it is not unheard of for them to become physically aggressive. Managers must endeavour to stay calm and in control. They must never rise to the challenge. It is a good idea to let these individuals finish their verbal onslaught before attempting to regain control of the meeting and focusing purely on the facts pertaining directly to them.

'The Professional Weeper' will use emotion to make managers feel guilty, or even apologetic. If the emotional outburst is merely an act, which subsequently fails, they can quickly become aggressive. Managers must remain focused and not weaken to the emotional onslaught. Having paper tissues available may demonstrate compassion but will be unlikely to alter the person's strategy.

'The Legal Eagle' will attempt to turn the interview into a courtroom. These individuals will likely deliver an entire dissertation on the intransigence of the management or organization. As with the 'counter attacker', managers need to let them say their piece before focusing solely on the facts relating to the individual or incident.

'The Artful Dodger' is very cunning and quick to think of defences such as, '*I wasn't there at the time!*' or, '*Well I sent the letter, didn't you get it?*' Managers must have all the facts available to them and give a clear message that they have all the facts. If any facts are not to hand, the interview should be suspended and then rescheduled at the earliest opportunity to ensure there is little room for the person to manipulate further.

In all instances of difficult interview subjects, the unequivocal management tool is *information*. Facts may be argued but they cannot be changed. If managers have all the facts to hand there will be little room for subordinates to argue with them. Being poorly prepared and without all the relevant information will afford interviewees an opportunity to use their manipulative tactics and compromise managers' control of the interview.

Although individuals employing such tactics will normally remain hostile on a verbal level, there is always a possibility that they could become physically violent.

Good communication skills are the key to managing any verbal interaction successfully, whether a meeting, interview or an encounter in or out of the workplace. Most physical assaults begin with a verbal exchange of some description. If the situation can be managed effectively at this level then the chances of a physical assault are reduced significantly. Understanding other people, observing them and identifying individual characteristics, and then communicating positively, is the most important facet to ensure the effective management of violence and aggression.

## INTERVIEW ARRANGEMENTS

When conducting interviews it is important to establish an open atmosphere that encourages positive communication. Traditionally, interviewers sit behind a desk, but this instantly presents a barrier between themselves and clients. Similarly, it is quite common for clients' chairs to be arranged to be lower, deliberately placing them at a psychological disadvantage. The following interview plans (Figure 5.3 A–D) are structured to achieve different results. The interviewer is on the left in all instances.

(A)

(B)

(C)

(D)

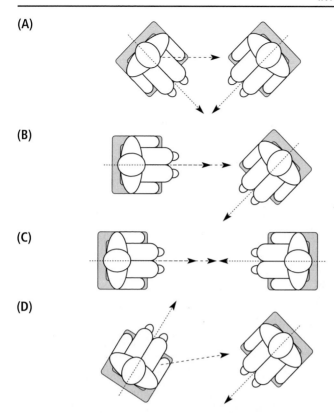

**Figure 5.3** (A) Open triangular formation. This establishes an informal and relaxed environment which encourages rapport. Places both parties on equal footing. (B) Direct body position. Establishes a position of control. Indicates that the interviewer wants straight answers to straight questions. Combined with gaze and reduced body and facial gestures, the subject will feel immense non-verbal pressure. This direct position can easily be attained from the open-triangular set-up by simply turning the chair to face subordinate. (C) Direct body position 2. This time both parties are directly facing each other. This can prove intimidating for the subordinate, applying even more non-verbal pressure. (D) Right angle position. The interviewer positioning the body at a right angle to the subject takes the pressure off the interview. This is a good position from which to ask potentially delicate or embarrassing questions, encouraging more open answers.

# Chapter 6

# RESPONSIBILITY AND ACCOUNTABILITY

## INTRODUCTION

Before using any defensive strategies, whether physical or verbal, it must be understood that everyone involved has to be accountable for their actions. This applies in any situation, whether in the workplace or in everyday life. Should anybody act inappropriately with the consequence of any physical (or psychological) detriment to others, they will be held accountable.

Every professional organization will have a policy concerning the use of physical force for defence or intervention purposes. The majority of employers will educate all new recruits as to the nature of any policy in operation, even if it only means giving them a copy of the text, and it is their responsibility to do so under Health and Safety legislation. Should an organization fail to do this, employees should endeavour to obtain the relevant information for themselves, although they are under no obligation to do so. Searching out relevant information, and making sure all information supplied is learnt, is simply good individual practice.

## USE OF PHYSICAL SELF-DEFENCE

In the clinical environment, staff are charged with a 'duty of care' to their clients and extra rules will normally apply. These will cater for many situations, which will be dictated by care plans and other factors. In a working or social environment, it is unacceptable to use any form of physical strike, kick or other blow, unless in an extreme self-defence or life-threatening situation. Even in these instances individuals will be held accountable for their actions. If the instance was so severe, with no other source of help, and no option but to strike back, individuals involved will take the necessary action, but only in the knowledge that they will be held responsible for their actions. Policies rarely cover such extreme instances.

Section 3 of the Criminal Law Act 1967 (16) states that, 'a person may use such force as is reasonable in the circumstances in the prevention of crime'. This article of law makes provision for interventions into an aggressive situation where there is an assault being committed, or the likelihood of an assault being committed. It is also true that the same reasonable force can be applied to individuals' self-defence. The key word is *reasonable*.

At the instant of an aggressive situation, individuals need to decide what response is actually deemed 'reasonable'. By use of the conflict resolution plan (see p. 29), combined with their own perceptions of the situation, individuals may formulate what they believe to be the right or necessary response. In extreme instances, for example where their life or the lives of others are in danger, extreme force may be required. Such force would be likely to injure, possibly seriously, an aggressor, but provided it could be justified that the force was necessary, and not excessive, it could still be deemed reasonable. In very extreme circumstances the use of lethal force could even be justified, but the anticipated consequences of its use have to be as severe, and the situation must be life-threatening, leaving no other option available.

'Excessive force' may be defined as, 'more force than was necessary to ensure personal safety or to ensure the safety of others'. Whatever force is required to ensure the safety of practitioners is reasonable, but once safety is assured no more force must be used. Additional force would be classed as excessive. The use of excessive force after safety has been assured simply cannot be justified and may even be seen as delivering punishment.

It is not always possible for practitioners or service-providers to escape without conflict, or to make a breakaway technique work for them. In these instances the use of strikes and blows may be acceptable, provided they are deployed only with reasonable force and they can be justified.

If employees adhere strictly to the guidelines laid down in policy, and the guidelines of common law, an organization will stand by them in any subsequent legal action. If employees stray from policy and use any unauthorized or non-recommended techniques, or excessive force, an organization will not be obliged to offer any support. The majority of such instances will result in an inquiry and, ultimately, either suspension or dismissal. Acts such as striking another person, client or co-worker, can potentially result in instant dismissal. Further to company actions there will always be the very real possibility of legal action by the other party or criminal proceedings by the police.

Criminal law applies when an offence is committed and the police make enquiries leading to a criminal charge, such as assault. This case is then passed to the Crown Prosecution Service, where it is assessed and a decision made as to whether to commit it to court. If found guilty of a criminal offence individuals may either be fined heavily, imprisoned or both.

Civil law operates when complainants decide to sue privately for compensation. If they have enough financial resources to fund a case, a solicitor will issue a court summons and prosecute through the County or High Courts. If individuals do not have sufficient funds to pursue the case, but do have a strong case, they may well receive Legal Aid for their action. Defendants will have to pay their own legal fees, plus the plaintiff's costs, if they lose. Although defendants may not face a jail sentence if found guilty, they can be fined very heavily or ordered to pay a financial sum in compensation. Any prosecution, civil or criminal, will place the defendant under considerable strain.

In the working environment if the force used to ensure personal safety was reasonable and in keeping with organizational policy, practitioners should be covered under 'vicarious liability', in which case any legal action will be diverted beyond them towards the organization. There will be provision within professional organizations for indemnity cover to deal with such incidents through the organization's regulated governing body or council.

If an extreme attack occurs outside the working environment, again, defenders must resort to Common Law and self-defence techniques. This may also apply within the working situation, where a defender may have no alternative but to strike out or resort to other self-defence strategies. As outlined in the work application, any action must be justifiable. In respect of self-defence, the law allows individuals the right to protect themselves against violence, or threatened violence, with whatever force or means are reasonably necessary. Another term often used is that of 'minimum force'. The words may be slightly different but the meaning should be considered the same. As in the work environment, to be safe, reasonable force should always be considered 'minimum force'.

In a defence situation, minimum force is enough force to enable the defender to escape, and *no more*. If a defender gains an advantage or an opportunity to escape, but having gained the upper hand decides to teach an aggressor a lesson, this would be considered as punishment and as 'excessive force'. The moment an opportunity for escape occurs, it must be taken.

Different individuals will interpret 'minimum force' to mean different things, allowing for confusion over what is acceptable and what is not. The reality is that some individuals may consider that no violence of any kind, even if used in self-defence, is acceptable. However, defensive techniques may be necessary, and if so, should be delivered with enough commitment to ensure they succeed. For some, that force may always be deemed excessive, but in the cold reality of a life-threatening confrontation it is not wise to deliver any technique without a degree of force.

The law and organizational policies are constantly changing and every organization has a duty to keep informed as to what is acceptable at any given time, and to pass that information to employees. Adhering to policies and law will provide a good degree of safety but transgressing the guidelines will leave individuals concerned extremely vulnerable. Ultimately, in any situation the consequences must be considered. All policy and procedures must be followed to the letter and any action undertaken must be done so in the knowledge that those involved will have to be accountable for their actions.

If it is necessary to use force, it should be reasonable, applicable, effective and justifiable, and delivered in the knowledge that it will nearly always have to be accounted for.

## 'NO-GO' AREAS OF THE BODY

When attempting any intervention or control type of technique there are certain areas of the body that should be avoided at all costs. These 'no-go' areas are illustrated in Figure 6.1.

It is always recommended to only ever hold or manipulate people by the limbs, never by the joints. There are always exceptions and professionals, with experience and skill, can readily control subjects by the joints in relative safety. This is only to be attempted in extreme situations, or once a level of proficiency has been achieved. Even then accidents can and do happen and it wise to remember that common sense minimizes risk.

The determination of 'extreme' needs to be established by practitioners in relation to the conflict resolution plan. Very few individuals would class themselves as professionals when dealing

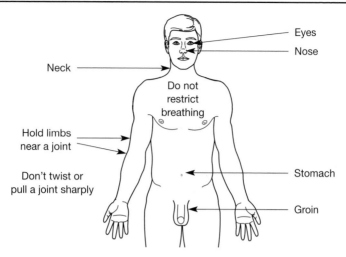

**Figure 6.1** 'No-go' areas of the body.

with violence and aggression, although many individuals are trained in such techniques. Skill level varies widely and the different impact factors (see p. 31) applying to different circumstances may negate the use of certain techniques and render others ineffective, regardless of ability or skill.

The use of pain compliance controls applied to the joints can, if effective, result in clients becoming more agitated through anger, fear or resentment. These feelings may serve to fuel their aggression further during the episode, or may fuel subsequent aggressive behaviour in the future. Regardless of the duty of care it should be considered that practitioners have elected to pursue a career in which their role is primarily to care for and enrich the lives of others. The safety and well-being of clients is of paramount importance and should not be forgotten, irrespective of any violent outburst, otherwise the entire principle of providing care becomes a mute exercise.

Certainly a situation that was life-threatening, for either practitioners or third parties, could be described as extreme, but the response needed must still be 'reasonable'. Practitioners need to be aware of the implications of attempting a control or strike to a vulnerable area of the body. If it is still necessary to apply such a strike, that is a decision to be made at that time, whilst being aware of the consequences.

Strikes need to be avoided, unless totally necessary, in which case they should be aimed at the limbs and never directed towards the head or spine areas. Any blow to an aggressor's body, particularly to vulnerable areas, such as the throat, spine or kidneys, can result in serious injury. Similarly, any blows to the head can cause impact damage to soft tissue areas, such as the eye or mouth, or concussive damage to the skull, including fractures.

Any pressure applied onto the chest may restrict the breathing, which can also result in harm, particularly if subjects end up face-down in a prone position. The danger in this situation will occur from the risk of 'positional asphyxia'. This is a condition that occurs when subjects cannot breathe, owing to their own bodyweight, either on its own or being held down in an attempt to control them, pressing down and pushing the stomach up into the diaphragm, consequently restricting the breathing. People can die of suffocation through positional asphyxia.

It should be noted that the risk of positional asphyxia is increased if subjects are obese, due to the increased size of the stomach being pushed upwards into the chest. Subjects lying face-down need to be placed into a recovery position as soon as it is practicable to do so.

Other important 'no-go' areas include the neck and the mouth. Restricting either can cause respiratory problems for subjects and as a consequence carry a significant risk. The Mental Health Act (1983) Code of Practice forbids any application of neckholds, clearly reinforcing the potential for injury.

In the heat of a conflict it may prove difficult to focus on policy and to adhere cleanly to guidelines and protocol, particularly if an incident is very intense and the risk of personal injury, or perceived risk of personal in injury, is high. However, even in such volatile circumstances it is vital to consider what techniques are being used and how exactly they are being applied, including specific areas of the subjects' body being targeted. Opportune application of an ethical technique can resolve a conflict very effectively but a momentary lapse, leading to a technique applied to a vulnerable area, may have serious consequences.

Chapter 7

# NON-AVERSIVE BREAKAWAY TECHNIQUES

## INTRODUCTION

Even a complete understanding of aggression management, combined with good communication skills, may sometimes still be not enough to avoid a physical confrontation.

In a physical confrontation there is normally an attacker and a defender. The defenders' main priority must be to escape. Standing and fighting could result in serious injury and the longer they spend with an attacker, the greater becomes the chance of injury. Defenders working in the clinical professions have responsibility for the safety of their clients, but if they are seriously injured themselves they will be unable to protect or assist anybody else.

Unless an individual is being physically restrained by an aggressor, it should be possible for them to attempt an escape. The exception to this occurs when an individual is cornered, with no obvious escape route. Being aware of surroundings and other people should serve to avoid this situation. As the majority of confrontations begin with a verbal exchange it is important for defenders to maintain a safe distance from a potential aggressor.

## PERSONAL SPACE

'Personal space' is a term used to describe the area immediately surrounding an individual. This area is normally recognized as a distance just beyond the length of an individual's own arms (Figure 7.1). Keeping aggressors beyond arm's length during a verbal exchange lessens the opportunity for them to grab hold of their victims, as they would have to step or reach forward to do so. Such a step or reach could be seen by defenders and they could either step back or block the attempted grab, but only if they were 'aware' (see p. 23) in the first instance. If aggressors were allowed to breach the area of personal space and get close it would be very easy for them to grab or strike their victims (Figure 7.2).

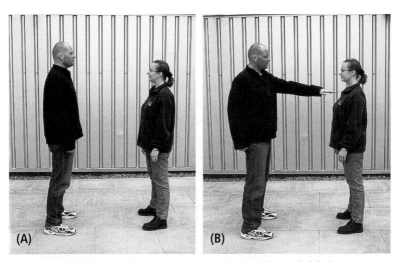

**Figure 7.1** (A) A good distance to preserve 'personal space'. (B) The same distance measured by length of arm.

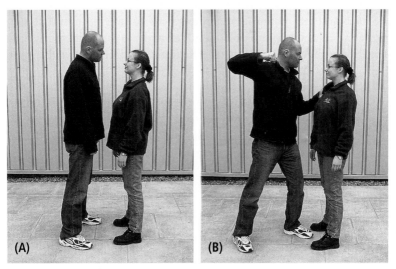

**Figure 7.2** (A) Aggressor far too close for practitioner to manage situation and to see or react to any possible attack. (B) At this range aggressor can easily strike or grab.

Although it is important to preserve personal space it is far better for practitioners to create a good 'reactionary gap' (Figure 7.3) between themselves and clients, ideally between two and four metres. Even having preserved the personal space zone, serious aggressors could cover that distance very quickly in a physical assault. A good reactionary gap is much harder to cross quickly and easier for defenders to work within.

Whilst a confrontation is at a verbal level defenders should automatically try and enhance communication. The use of 'open' hand gestures at this stage will automatically place their hands between them and an attacker, providing a natural barrier and also an advantage should a block be required. Should attackers attempt a grab or strike they will have to get past the defenders' hands first in order to do so. Similarly, a desk or chair can provide a good natural barrier for defenders to stand behind if deemed necessary.

Without 'awareness' it is impossible to identify a potential threat. Assuming individuals are aware, and have identified a threat, their first priority must be to escape or to seek assistance. If this is not possible then they must try and talk to aggressors, preserving the reactionary gap while doing so. At this stage, awareness is still vitally important in order to identify any opportunities for escape, or in order to react to a physical attack.

Posture is of an equal importance when preparing to respond to a physical threat. Balance and stability are required for effective defence and any potential defenders need to take a neutral stance, with the feet approximately shoulder-width apart and the weight evenly distributed. Should too much weight be placed over either foot,

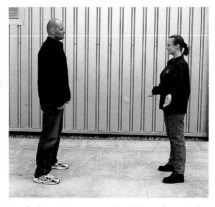

**Figure 7.3** A good, safe 'reactionary gap', although not always practicable, or achievable.

defenders instantly become unbalanced and could easily be pushed over. Even weight distribution also enables them to move readily in any direction without first having to shift the bodyweight to do so.

Should defenders have their hands full, or in their pockets, they would be unable to block any grab or strike effectively. If items are being carried, they should be carefully placed down, without leaving a defensive vulnerability. If a situation suddenly becomes violent then any items carried could simply be dropped. Items can be replaced, people cannot! It should also be considered that any items carried could be picked up and used as potential weapons by aggressors – either to strike with or to be thrown.

Taking all the relevant precautions and endeavouring to communicate with aggressors unfortunately does not guarantee that they will not become physically violent. A natural reaction is for aggressors to grab hold of and restrain their victims. Such a grab may preceed a striking technique, or merely enable them to gain control of defenders for other purposes. In the instance of a grab, victims must resist the urge to strike out in defence.

Striking out and hitting clients is to be considered only ever as a last resort, when there is genuine fear for the practitioners' personal safety or survival. Striking techniques are severely frowned upon and, considering the applicable policies, ethics and duty of care, should only ever be considered if there is no other alternative to ensure safety. Should practitioners strike out and hit an attacker it could potentially be seen as an assault – therefore such action has to be totally justifiable. Any unjustifiable and unnecessary assault in the workplace will almost automatically result in dismissal and/or court proceedings.

Should a strike be used, it must be justified as reasonable in the circumstances and excessive force must not be used. Reasonable force (see p. 67) would be accepted as enough force to enable escape and/or to ensure personal safety. Anything beyond this would be deemed as excessive force and cannot be justified.

If struck, it is also possible that aggressors will not be sufficiently harmed or deterred from their attack, and having been angered further, may strike back even harder. In this instance there is the possibility of defenders being seriously injured. Serious consideration needs to be given to the use of any striking technique, particularly to the consequences of their use, and therefore the proper use of breakaway techniques may provide a more reasonable and ethical solution.

The non-aversive breakaway techniques illustrated in this chapter are designed to get potential victims away from aggressors without the need for any striking techniques. They are all proven, but in order to be called upon in an emergency they must not only be learnt but also practised periodically.

## LEARNING PRACTICAL TECHNIQUES

**Important note**

This work is intended to provide a learning resource or review package for students who have already attended a training course. It is a reference segment, and is *not* intended as a self-instruction programme. No responsibility can be accepted for any incident or situation that may arise from individuals attempting self-tuition from this work.

It is not easy to learn physical defence movements or breakaway techniques from illustrations in a book, from a film or from any other such limited format. Works such as this are designed for review purposes for students or practitioners who are attending, or who have already attended, a structured training programme. The illustration of practical techniques can also enable students to reaffirm their skills or to identify any flaws in their methods.

To maintain operational proficiency and to ensure that clear understanding is achieved, even if only used as a review tool, the steps shown must be followed exactly as illustrated, and the techniques practised repeatedly as described.

All the moves illustrated are tried and tested, utilized by practitioners in both the Trust and private sectors. They are proven in application, provided they are learnt correctly and practised regularly. Unfortunately, in a relaxed practice situation it is easy to believe that a technique has been learnt, when in truth it requires further repetition in order for it to be called upon in an emergency. Similarly, a practice scenario is not a true representation of a real encounter. There is no pressure on either defenders or aggressors to ensure success and they will not be experiencing true emotions, such as fear or panic. Put simply, there is no real threat or genuine survival instinct by which to measure the validity of the technique.

It is important that students believe in the technique and do not become disheartened if progress is slow or their practice partner endeavours to be too clever or difficult for them. Regardless of the situation, real attackers generally expect to succeed in their assaults, or certainly will not have considered failure. They do not anticipate any difficulty or serious resistance. If aggressors expected any serious resistance, it is unlikely that they would attack in the first place.

Ultimately, defenders have the 'element of surprise' in their favour, which is a significant advantage that is not present unless the encounter is real.

The techniques included are not structured as a course, but follow the structure most commonly facilitated. Therefore, for the best results it is suggested that only one hour at a time is allocated for review, with at least one day's break between sessions. Only one or two techniques should be attempted per session, which should then be practised solidly for that full session, and then reviewed again at the beginning of each subsequent hour of review. Reviewing in this way encourages a cumulative learning process. Practice between sessions is also beneficial.

All physical techniques need to be practised slowly and with a compliant partner, who understands what is trying to be achieved. There are certain training preparations that need to be observed to ensure safety and that the moves are learnt correctly.

The first thing to consider is location. An area of clear space with an even floor is vital. Sports facilities or a large clear garden are ideal; a living room is not. Those participating should wear flat shoes, loose clothing and remove all jewellery. Although the techniques should be practised slowly, it is necessary to undertake some form of light warm-up exercises, possibly including some low-intensity stretching, to prepare the body for practice. As no two people are alike it is not possible to recommend a general programme of exercises that would be suited to all prospective participants. Professional advice should be sought from a suitably qualified physical trainer, in conjunction with the individuals' own GPs, to ensure an appropriate warm-up programme is implemented for everyone concerned.

No warm-up information is provided in this text because the work is intended solely for review and the illustration of such movements would imply that it would be possible to self-teach the techniques from a book. Equally, to meet the needs of every individual in respect of exercises would be an unrealistic undertaking.

It should be understood that the techniques must be practised with both sides, that is, both left- and right-handed, although only one side is illustrated in the text. Practitioners must be able to use breakaway techniques from either hand in order to be completely effective. It is not unknown for people to practice a defensive technique using only the left hand and then to find themselves unable to apply the movement with the right.

Before reviewing the following techniques a final consideration is that there is *no substitute for proper tuition*. The illustrations provide an excellent study aid to accompany a course or for review purposes, and whilst in certain circumstances it may prove possible to learn the movements from the text, words and pictures are not a reasonable substitute for professional tuition in a course environment. There are many specialist trainers providing comprehensive courses in breakaway techniques and associated matters for clinical application. Most schools of health studies will have in place programmes and contact details for suitably qualified professional trainers.

## MEDICAL IMPLICATIONS

All the techniques illustrated are non-aversive and low intensity, and are designed to minimize totally the risk of any injury to either practitioners or clients. However, it should be understood and accepted that in any physical activity there is always some risk, no matter how slight, of injury. The movements should offer little chance of any injury, but as the weight, size and age gap widens there may be a low risk of potential minor injuries. An extreme example would be if a young, strong practitioner applied a technique with force against an elderly or infirm client. For reference, each technique is accompanied by a 'Medical implications' box, which outlines any possible injury that may be resultant from its application.

The medical implications stated by no means form a comprehensive or exhaustive list, they are merely the most likely potential injuries that could occur in extreme circumstances. The techniques are the most non-aversive available, offering minimum risk potential for injury, but in application, or indeed in practice, risk can never be ruled out completely. Similarly, it is also possible that in extreme circumstances during application or practice, injuries other than those outlined could be sustained. This further supports the need for all training to be facilitated only in a controlled and managed environment, and that any real 'in service' application should be undertaken with due care and consideration.

## NON-AVERSIVE BREAKAWAY TECHNIQUES

None of the techniques included are dependent on physical strength or size to be effective, but they do rely on the movement of body weight. Should practitioners merely attempt to pull themselves free of a restraint without stepping away and subsequently using their body weight, they will be unlikely to succeed. Combining the techniques shown with a positive step and transference of weight will ensure a far greater chance of success.

Although photographs can illustrate movements, it is difficult to convey the necessary timing. To ensure a greater understanding of the mechanics is acquired, all the accompanying notes should be observed before practice.

## Wrist grabs

Although sometimes perceived as a low-intensity threat, wrist grabs allow aggressors to restrain the movement of practitioners and can precede a punch or other similar strike. Equally, whilst held, practitioners cannot withdraw and may be unable to summon assistance. The threat may be seen as low but it can easily escalate and consequently escape is vital, but must be low-intensity and non-aversive.

## FRONTAL STRAIGHT-ON WRIST GRAB

This is used solely to facilitate escape from an aggressor.

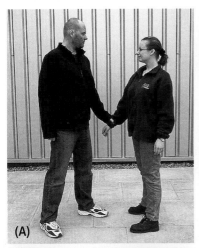 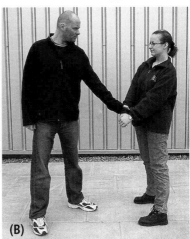

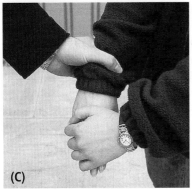

**Figure 7.4** (A) Aggressor (on left) grabs defender's wrist straight on (left to right or right to left). (B) Defender firmly clasps the restrained hand with her free hand. (C) Close-up of (B) showing defender clasping trapped hand with her free hand.

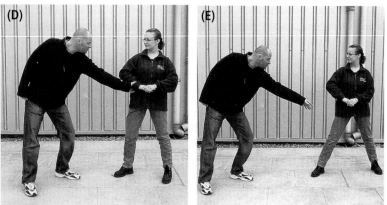

**Figure 7.4** (D) Defender pulls trapped hand close to her body, whilst beginning to step away and overextending the aggressor. (E) Defender continues positive step to pull completely clear whilst establishing a good reactionary gap.

> ### Medical implications
> Technique is very low risk but in extreme circumstances there may be adverse pressure on aggressor's fingers, wrist or shoulder. Resultant injury is unlikely but there is possibility of sprain or dislocation.

## FRONTAL DIAGONAL WRIST GRAB

### Very important

The step utilized in all the techniques illustrated *must* be positive and be as long as is reasonably practicable to execute. A decisive, purposeful step will ensure that escape is achieved and will help to displace an aggressor's posture (notice the line of the aggressor's shoulder in Figure 7.5(E)). A weak, short or casual step is unlikely to achieve an effective escape as it will not employ an effective transfer of the defender's bodyweight through an aggressor's grasp. A short step will still leave defenders within an aggressor's reach and not facilitate the maximum efficiency of the technique. A long step will shift the defender's bodyweight but will also facilitate resumption of a useable reactionary gap (Figure 7.6).

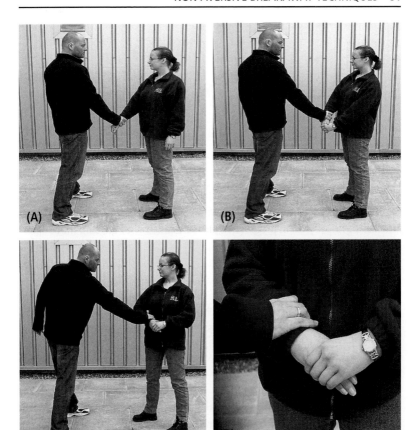

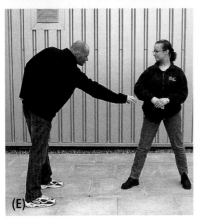

**Figure 7.5** (A) Aggressor (on left) grabs defender's wrist diagonally across the body (left to left, or right to right). (B) Defender grabs the trapped hand with her free hand. (C) Defender begins to step away from aggressor, with a positive step, whilst pulling hands close into her body. (D) Close-up of (C) showing defender hand position, close into her body. (E) Defender continues long, decisive step away, whilst continuing to pull trapped hand close to her body and away from the aggressor.

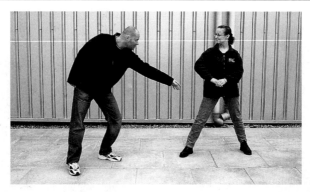

**Figure 7.6** Defender continues step, whilst pulling her hand away past the attacker's grasp, by using progressive pressure timed with the step (not snatching the hand away!).

## Medical implications

Low risk but if applied with extreme vigour there may be adverse pressure applied on aggressors' fingers, wrists or shoulders. Resultant injury is unlikely but there is a possibility of sprain or dislocation.

### Important note

The weakest part of any individual's grasp is where the fingers meet the thumb. This is the point where the trapped hand must be pulled against, and through, to achieve a successful escape. Pulling against the hand or wrist will not achieve an escape but could also possibly result in injury to an aggressor. This method should be applied to *all* wrist grab escapes using the stepping principle.

The principle of pulling through a grasp whilst moving the body-weight away from an opponent may be applied to any single-wrist grab (unless control is required – see 'Front diagonal wrist grab 2' below). The direction of step and pull may change but the principle always remains the same.

The pull and step must be extremely positive and timed together, using total commitment. Attempting to yank the hand free sharply will, in most cases, fail to work. Similarly, stepping first and then trying to pull the hand free will also fail, as will trying to pull the hand free before stepping. The key to success is the timed movement of bodyweight combined with the technique of pulling against the weakest part of the grasp.

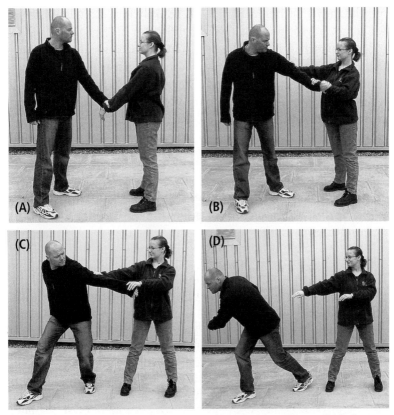

**Figure 7.7** (A) Aggressor (on left) grabs defenders wrist diagonally (left to left or right to right). (B) Defender rotates the trapped wrist in an inside-to-out direction with palm face down and grabs the attacking wrist, whilst applying pressure with her free hand on the aggressor's upper arm, just above the elbow joint. (Note: If the attacker had hold of the right wrist the rotation would be in a clockwise direction. If the left wrist was being held the rotation would be anti-clockwise.) (C) By keeping hold of the wrist and stepping into the aggressor, whilst pushing firmly onto the upper arm, momentary control can be achieved if needed. (D) A more assertive step, combined with a positive push-away can serve to push the aggressor away and create a safe gap.

## FRONT DIAGONAL WRIST GRAB 2

This defence against the same grab permits a greater degree of safety and, whilst slightly more complicated, may be used to gain control of an aggressor if needed (Figure 7.7).

Although control is achieved it is unlikely that it can be sustained for long and so it is not recommended for this purpose, merely to gain momentary control whilst summoning assistance. Similarly, the push-away method can be seriously affected by relevant impact factors, as outlined in the conflict resolution plan (see p. 29). Both techniques can be effective but must be practised to ensure efficiency and even then only used with caution.

> ### Medical implications
> Very low risk with push-away application. Minimal potential for sprained wrists or shoulders if the subject is weak or infirm. Extreme application could result in dislocation. Control technique carries low risk, with similar minimal injury potential.

## DIAGONAL WRIST GRAB CONTROL

### Very important
This technique (Figure 7.8) is designed solely to gain control in extreme instances of threat or danger. It is very aversive and consequently *must* be justifiable. The technique is not ratified for general application. It must also be considered whether such a method of control is contrary to organizational policy or the duty of care.

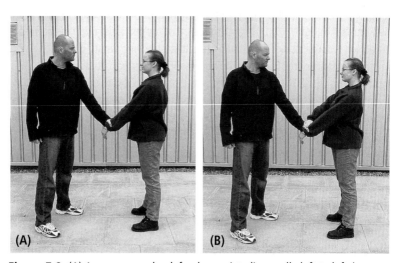

**Figure 7.8** (A) Aggressor grabs defenders wrist, diagonally left to left (or right to right). (B) Defender places free hand firmly on the back of the attacking hand, securing it in place.

The technique can be held at this position (Figure 7.8(F)) in order to gain an element of control. However, it is not recommended to try and use this as a restraining move other than for a few seconds whilst summoning assistance. If an aggressor is extremely hostile and help is

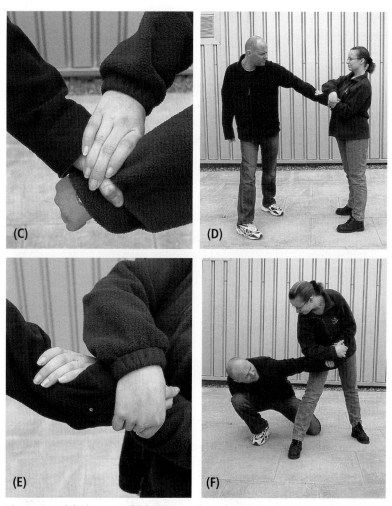

**Figure 7.8** (C) Close-up of (B) showing the subject's hand being secured by the defender's free hand. (D) Defender now rotates trapped wrist in an inside-to-out motion (in the example counter-clockwise) and grabs hold of the attacking wrist, still holding the hand firmly in place. (E) Close up of (D) showing the wrist rotation and grab, whilst still securing the attacking hand. (F) Defender now steps across the subject and allows the elbow of the controlling hand to connect firmly with the subject's elbow, forcing them into a controlled position.

not forthcoming then an attempted restrain could endanger practitioners further should their opponents be strong enough to escape.

### Medical implications

High risk – vigorous or uncontrolled application may result in sprained, dislocated or broken wrists or shoulders, particularly if subjects are resistant,
or if they are weak or infirm. The technique can be used very effectively
without inflicting any injury at all, provided it is practised extensively and a
high level of proficiency is attained. Only to be used with caution and with
justification.

## DOUBLE-HANDED WRIST GRAB 1

This technique involves two hands onto one (Figure 7.9).

### Medical implications

Very, very low risk, carrying little potential for injury. In very extreme
instances there is the possibility of sprained or dislocated fingers, wrists or
shoulders.

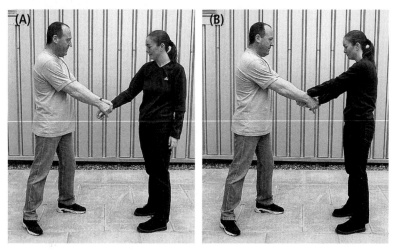

**Figure 7.9** (A) Aggressor (on left) grabs defender's single wrist with both
hands. (B) Defender reaches between aggressor's hands and firmly grabs hold
of her trapped hand.

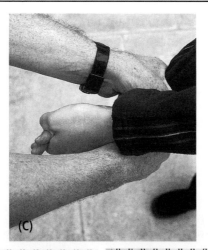

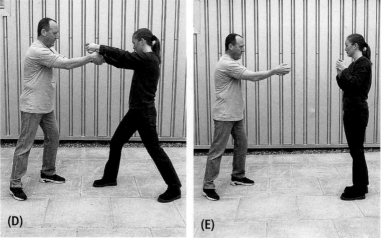

**Figure 7.9** (C) Close up of (B) showing defender grabbing her own trapped hand firmly. (D) Defender now begins to step positively backwards whilst at the same time pulling both hands upwards. (E) Defender continues step back, bringing feet together and hands to her body, completing the technique and establishing a good reactionary gap.

## DOUBLE-HANDED WRIST GRAB 2

This manoeuvre is for a single wrist to single wrist grab defence (Figure 7.10). The technique relies very much on a fluid motion and therefore requires practice. In a real application this fluidity, combined with the element of surprise, should ensure success. Attempts to snatch the hands away should be avoided.

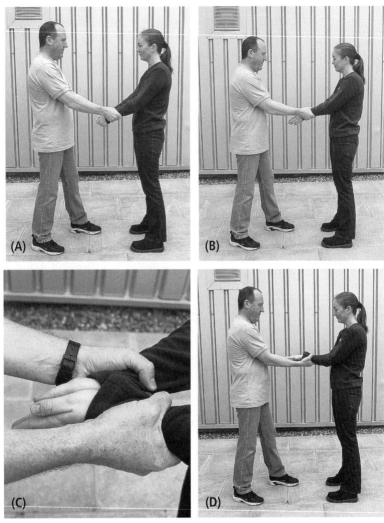

**Figure 7.10** (A) Aggressor (on left) grabs hold of each of the subject's wrists, one hand to each wrist. (B) Defender brings both her hands together in a clapping-type motion. (C) Close-up of (B) – defender brings her hands together palm to palm. (D) Defender now opens her hands out, palms facing up, whilst still keeping them together.

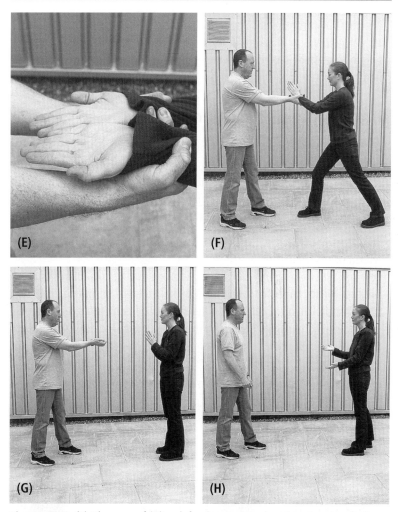

**Figure 7.10** (E) Close-up of (D) – defender opening hands out, palms facing upwards, keeping hands together. (F) Defender now steps back away from aggressor, closing hands back together and pulling them upwards, towards herself. (G) Defender continues her step away to complete technique and re-establish a good reactionary gap. (H) Defender maintains good distance and resumes communication whilst using open hand gestures.

### Medical implications

Very, very low risk. In severe instances of misapplied technique against an infirm or resistant subject there may potentially be sprained or dislocated fingers, wrists or shoulders.

## SINGLE-HANDED CLOTHING GRAB

This technique (Figure 7.11) is purely a breakaway technique and may only be used for the clothing grab. If an aggressor attacks with the left hand (as illustrated) defenders must secure the grab with the left hand also. If the attack is with the right hand then defenders must use the right hand to secure the grasp.

### Medical implications

Low risk. Possible injury in extreme, vigorous application could occur to subjects' wrists, fingers or shoulders. Minimal potential of sprain or dislocation. Destabilizing aggressors during disengagement could, in extreme instances, result in them stumbling or falling, which could result in other potential minor injury.

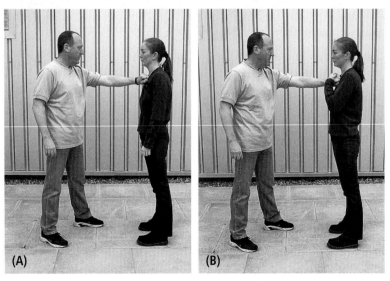

(A)      (B)

**Figure 7.11** (A) Aggressor (on left) grabs defender by the shirt. (B) Defender secures the attacking hand with her opposite free hand.

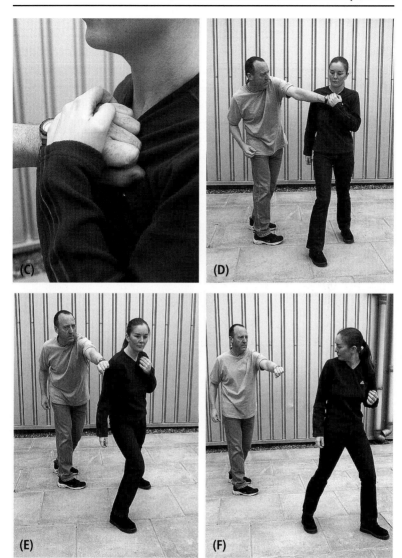

**Figure 7.11** (C) Close-up of (B) showing defender securing the attacking hand with her opposite free hand. (D) Defender now steps sharply across the front of the aggressor (from outside the attacking arm), enabling her shoulder to connect with the attacking arm and overextend the aggressor. (E) The defender continues her step, using her shoulder to completely disengage the attacker. (F) Defender continues to step away and escape, whilst maintaining visual contact with the subject.

## SINGLE-HANDED CLOTHING GRAB 2

This technique (Figure 7.12) includes an application for frontal choke. It is an optional technique following the principles outlined in the 'Single-handed clothing grab 1', but is more effective, allowing for an escape from a choke and also providing an option for control of aggressors. Control can readily be achieved but is only designed as a temporary measure, to be used to gain a momentary advantage or to summon assistance. It is not advised to attempt control as a final solution. Disengagement is a more realistic goal.

### Medical implications
Low risk, but in extreme, vigorous application there is potential for sprains or dislocation of subjects' wrists, fingers or shoulder joints.

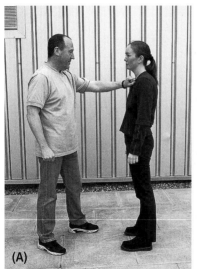 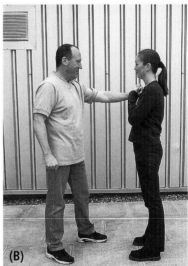

**Figure 7.12** (A) Aggressor grabs the defender with one hand by the shirt or neck. (B) Defender secures the grab tightly with her opposite free hand. (Following the principles outlined in Figure 7.11, parts (A) to (C)).

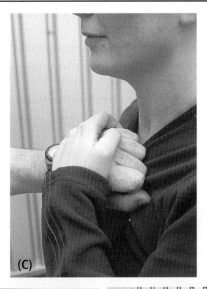

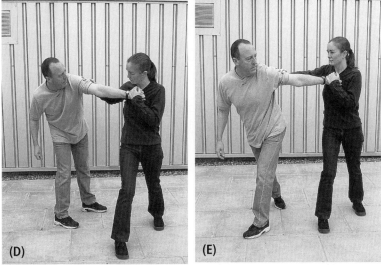

**Figure 7.12** (C) Close-up of (B), showing defender securing the attacker's hand with her opposite free hand (left to left). (D) Defender steps across the front of the attacker from the outside of the attacking arm whilst applying pressure with the palm of her free hand onto the attacker's upper arm, above the shoulder joint. (E) Increased pressure allows for a short-term control technique. Pushing away hard would enable a disengagement.

## SINGLE-HANDED CLOTHING GRAB 3

This manoeuvre (Figure 7.13) is a progression of the original technique as outlined earlier in Figure 7.11, only allowing for more pressure to be applied by defenders in the instance of a significant difference in size and weight between the two subjects. The same principle applies as in the original technique shown in Figure 7.11 – if an attacker grabs with the left hand then defenders must also secure with the left hand. Equally, if the attack is made with the right hand, defenders must also use the right hand.

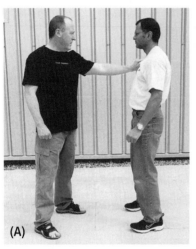

(A)

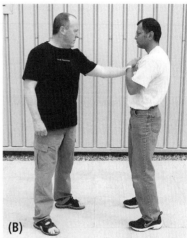

(B)

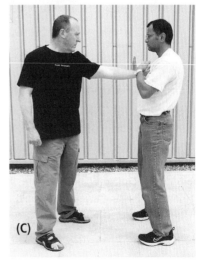

(C)

**Figure 7.13** (A) Aggressor (on left) grabs defender by the shirt. (B) Defender secures attacking hand with his opposite free hand. (C) Defender now pushes his free hand firmly against the attacker's wrist whilst preparing to step.

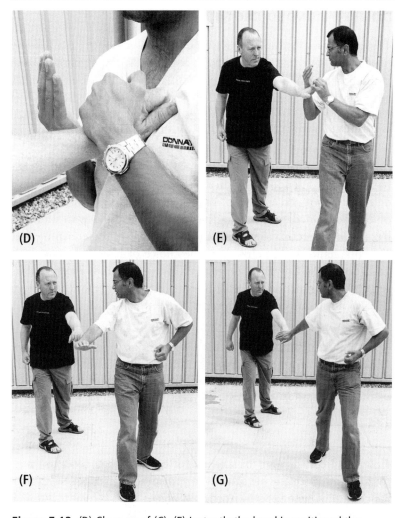

**Figure 7.13** (D) Close-up of (C). (E) Instantly the hand is positioned the defender steps positively from the outside, pushing the attacking hand through and away, using a strong turn of the hip. (F) The defender continues his long step to totally disengage the aggressor. (G) Defender steps through to get clear and establish a good reactionary gap whilst still keeping good eye contact on the subject.

### Medical implications

Low-intensity and low risk, but in extreme instances, if applied with excess vigour, the technique could possibly result in sprained wrists, fingers or dislocated shoulders.

## DOUBLE-HANDED CLOTHING GRAB 1

This technique (Figure 7.14) is designed to disengage from a double-handed clothing grab or choke from the front. If dealing with a choke it should be recognized that the potential threat is instantly greater and therefore a heightened sense of purpose must be employed. This would also apply to the single-handed choke as outlined earlier (see Figure 7.12). In a real application, undue hesitancy in either technique could prove extremely hazardous to the practitioner's safety.

This technique is ambidextrous and may be applied with either hand by the defender. The direction used may be decided by the defender's own perceptions of their personal strength in either arm or by the immediate surroundings. If there were a wall or other hazardous object in the immediate vicinity it may determine that only one hand could be used, as the choice of hand will automatically determine the direction taken. The technique is illustrated as separate movements but once learnt, like all those in the text, it should run smoothly together as one movement.

### Medical implications

Low risk, but in extreme circumstances subjects could suffer from sprains or dislocations of the wrists, fingers or shoulders. In very extreme instances, owing to balance displacement, subjects could also fall over, which may result in other minor injury.

**Figure 7.14** (A) Aggressor (on left) grabs defender with both hands by the shirt. (B) Defender places her arm in a downward motion between the attacker's arms, close to her own body, allowing her wrist to come to rest under the attacker's wrist and her elbow to rest on top of the attacker's other wrist. (C) Defender now straightens her arm, pressing her elbow downwards and her wrist upwards until her forearm is vertical, applying adverse pressure onto aggressor's wrists. (D) Defender steps across her own body from the outside, using her free arm and movement of her bodyweight to apply pressure onto the aggressor's arms, which are now vulnerable due to his twisted and compromised posture. (E) Continuing her step, whilst continuing to apply pressure to the aggressor's arms, will enable a complete disengagement.

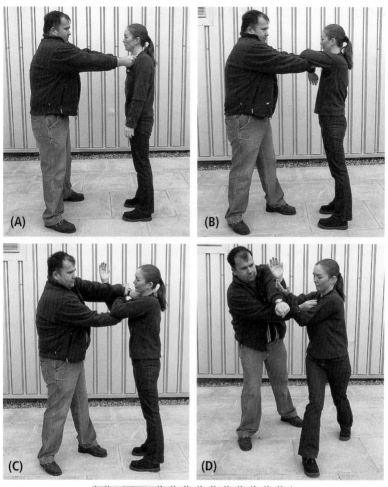

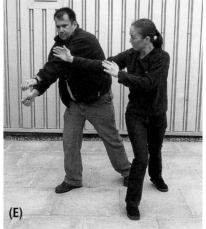

## DOUBLE-HANDED CLOTHING GRAB 2

This technique (Figure 7.15) offers a simple alternative to double-handed clothing grab 1. Although the term 'chest' is cited in the figure legend, consideration must be given to the subjects' gender and physical stature. In a choking scenario, target selection may be restricted through perceived threat but an effective area in which to apply pressure would be high on the chest, below the collar bone, or to the centre of the chest, if appropriate. Experience and common sense at the time will help to determine the most suitable region to use.

### Medical implications
Very, very low risk. In extreme instances subjects may receive adverse pressure to the fingers, wrists or shoulders, resulting in minimal potential for sprains or dislocations. Consideration must be given to whereabouts pressure is applied to the subject's chest, particularly if female. Excessive pressure against a poorly selected target could, in extreme instances, potentially result in temporary breathing difficulty and/or fracture to ribs, clavical or sternum.

## FRONTAL HAIR GRAB

The principle for dealing with a frontal hair grab (Figure 7.16) is exactly the same as that used for dealing with a frontal clothing grab or choke (see p. 92). The application of downward pressure onto the attacking hand helps to ease the pain of the hair pull by restricting the movement of an aggressor's hand. Hard downward pressure will in some instances also compact aggressors' knuckles, causing considerable pain. This may also cause them to release their grip.

Defenders may also find it effective to flex the knees as they apply the downward pressure, as this will automatically lower the centre of gravity and instantly increase their stability, decreasing the chance of being pulled forward, or over, by the hair.

The techniques need to be applied quickly in order to maintain control of balance and avoid aggressors gaining enough leverage to pull defenders downwards.

If an aggressor grabs with the left hand, defenders must apply pressure with the left hand also, following the principles employed for the single-handed clothing grab (see p. 92).

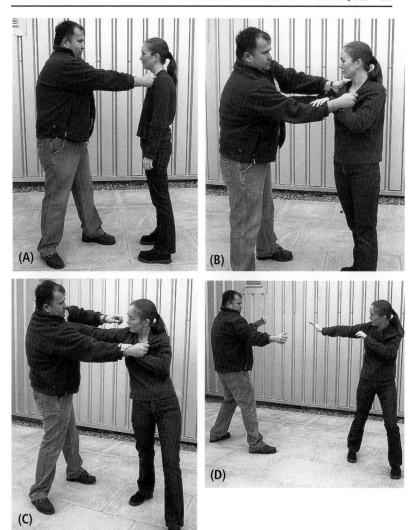

**Figure 7.15** (A) Aggressor (on left) grabs the defender by the shirt with both hands. (B) Defender brings her hands upwards between the aggressor's arms, pushing her leading palm into the aggressor's chest, whilst pushing the aggressor's arm outwards with her other hand. (Note: The term 'leading arm' is used to describe the same arm that is in relation to the leading or forward leg, or the leg that is to become the leading or forward leg.) (C) Defender now flexes her knees in order to achieve greater balance, whilst adopting a solid stance and twisting her hips away from the aggressor, pushing the palm of her leading hand into the attacker's chest and pushing his other hand clear. (D) Defender must move away quickly, without compromising stance or posture and achieve a reactionary gap.

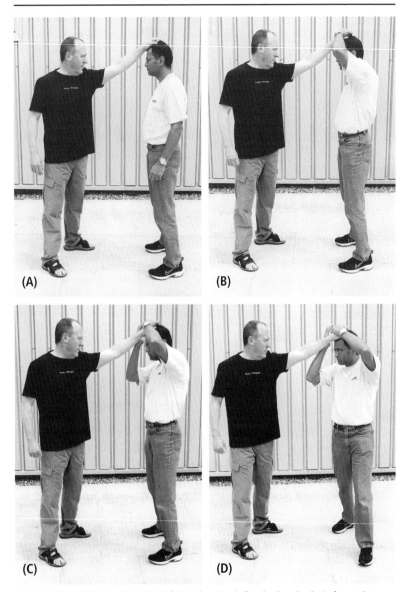

**Figure 7.16** (A) Attacker (on left) grabs the defender by the hair from the front with one hand. (B) Defender places opposite free hand firmly on top of the attacking hand and applies firm downward pressure. (C) Defender now applies pressure with opposite hand to the attacker's wrist, whilst preparing to step instantaneously across the front of the aggressor, from outside the attacking arm. (D) Defender instantly steps whilst still applying pressure and starts to disengage the aggressor.

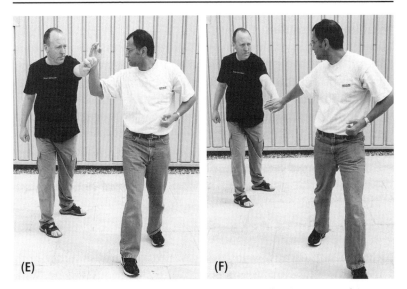

**Figure 7.16** (E) Continuing the step, whilst pushing firmly against, and through, the attacker's wrist will ensure the disengagement is successful. (F) A further step creates a good reactionary gap, but eye contact must still be maintained.

Note that the defensive breakaway techniques described for the single-handed choke, clothing or hair grabs all require that the stepping movement is employed from outside the attacking arm, across the front of an aggressor's body. If used in the other direction the technique will fail, leaving defenders in an extremely vulnerable position.

A strong hair grab will provide aggressors with leverage from which to control defenders while they strike them or pull them to the floor. This determines that a positive defence must be used, although consideration must always be given to the justification of any technique or target selected. Pressure should only be applied to the elbow in extreme instances, where the threat is perceived strongest and the application most justified. Pushing with the palm of the hand will achieve the necessary results in the majority of applications. The use of a strike with the forearm can be justified in extreme instances but carries a considerable risk of injury to aggressors.

## Medical implications

Low risk if technique is applied with the palm, pushing against the arm. In extreme instances there is potential for sprains or dislocations of fingers, wrists or shoulders. Hard pressure of hand onto an aggressor's semi-closed hand may, again in extreme instances, lead to possible fractures of the fingers or damage to the finger joints. Strongly applied strikes with the forearm to an aggressor's elbow carries a medium risk, potentially causing damage to the joint through overextension or through the impact of the strike. The risk of long-term damage from such a strike is minimal.

## REAR SHOULDER GRAB

Although initially a low-intensity attack, the rear shoulder grab (Figure 7.17) may easily progress into a more serious assault. With any rear grab, practitioners are at an instant disadvantage and time is an important factor, necessitating a quick response.

The sweeping motion with the arm *must* be very exaggerated, allowing the shoulder joint to rotate and therefore loosening an aggressor's grip. The sweeping motion is deployed with the same arm in relation to the shoulder grabbed and must be in a rearward direction (that is, if the right shoulder is grabbed, as illustrated, the arm/shoulder sweep is clockwise in direction – rearward. If it were a left-handed attack the rotation would be counter-clockwise – still rearward.)

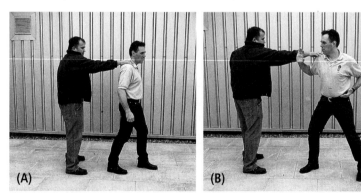

**(A)**　　　　**(B)**

**Figure 7.17**  (A) Aggressor (on left) grabs the defender by the shoulder from behind. (B) Defender steps away from aggressor, rotating away from the grabbing hand through a full 180°. Whilst executing the turn he also uses his arm in a large sweeping motion to disengage the grab.

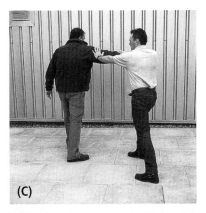

(C)

**Figure 7.17** (C) The turn and the step is completed, enabling the defender to readily push the aggressor away with both hands.

---

**Medical implications**
Very low risk, but the potential threat is high. In extreme instances subjects may sprain or dislocate fingers, wrists or shoulders.

---

## REAR CHOKE

A rear choke is a commonly used assault that carries a very high risk potential for defenders. It is not an attack that lends itself readily to easy defence techniques that may be assimilated on a short course or through a text.

The following technique (Figure 7.18) is not designed as a defensive escape technique. It is intended as a realistic movement to protect defenders from quickly being choked unconscious and to afford them an opportunity to summon assistance or gain time to think. It is a technique that is achievable without endangering practitioners further and has the potential to facilitate an escape, although such an escape would probably require a strike to be used and therefore it cannot be described as 'non-aversive'.

The technique will normally finish at the move shown in Figure 7.18(C), however, an opportunity may arise to step away, as shown in Figure 7.18(D). Equally, an opportunity may be created, once defenders are in a more stable position, as shown in Figure 7.18(C), by use of the elbow to strike an aggressor hard in the side of the body, causing a momentary distraction and an opportunity to escape. Any such strike can normally be reasonably justified in such a dangerous attack, although any elbow strike delivered must be done so with enough force to ensure that the escape opportunity arises and an aggressor is not merely further enraged. An elbow strike of the type required, as with all physical techniques, can normally only be learnt through a professional training programme.

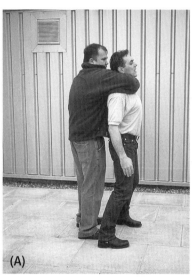

(A)

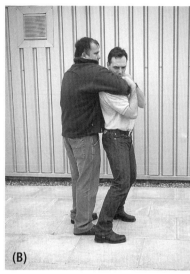

(B)

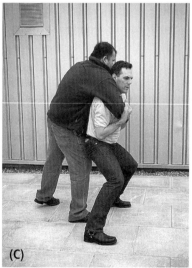

(C)

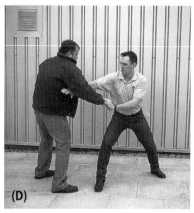

(D)

## Medical implications

Extremely low risk. No reasonable risk of injury to aggressors is anticipated unless an elbow strike is used. A strongly delivered elbow strike to the ribs could potentially crack or break the ribs. The implication of an aggressor's attack is that the defender could be choked unconscious or to death.

**Figure 7.18** (A) Aggressor (on left) applies a rear choke. (B) First priority for the defender is to protect the airway to avoid choking, by using both hands pulling downwards on the aggressor's arm and tucking the chin into the gap at the aggressor's elbow. (C) To avoid being thrown and to keep the airway free the defender *must immediately* widen the stance and drop the weight by bending the knees, whilst keeping both feet flat on the ground and the back perfectly straight. This may serve momentarily to displace the aggressor's balance, allowing the defender breathing space and a possibility to then either attempt to reason with the aggressor or to shout for assistance. (D) Should a gap open out because the aggressor's balance is briefly displaced it may be possible for the defender to stop and turn out of the choke, in a direction away from the choking arm.

# Chapter 8

# PHYSICAL INTERVENTIONS

## INTRODUCTION

In extreme circumstances it may become necessary for practitioners to control aggressive individuals, or to eject them from the establishment, in order to preserve the environment or the safety of others within it. Traditional 'control and restraint' (C&R) techniques have always proved extremely effective through the application of pressure against aggressors' joints, resulting in pain and compliance.

An inherent problem with these conventional techniques is that people have different pain thresholds and often cannot feel the technique working owing to adrenalin or being under the influence of alcohol or drugs, prescribed or otherwise. The principle of these techniques is to apply pressure to weak points, but as resistance builds it necessitates the application of more pressure. This can readily lead to injury and in a clinical environment this can lead to an inquiry and possible disciplinary action.

## ANOTHER WAY

Should a situation arise whereby an individual needs controlling or removing, the first priority must be to gain assistance. It is not recommended that any form of intervention be attempted without some form of help or back-up. If at all possible it is better to secure the environment without any form of physical intervention being attempted until there are enough people present to perform the technique effectively. As this is not always achievable, and help is not always readily to hand, the following technique (Figure 8.1) provides a possible solution.

The technique is appropriate for almost any workplace application, including, if used in accordance with policy and training, for
clinical use. There are other possibilities, but few that will ensure the
desired results with such minimal risk of injury to either party.
Instead of applying pressure to the joints, the technique works by
controlling the major limbs. Control is harder to achieve when
working with limbs, especially with a large or physically strong
opponent, and so a higher degree of proficiency is necessary to
ensure success with this technique. Achieving this requires extensive
practice and repetition.

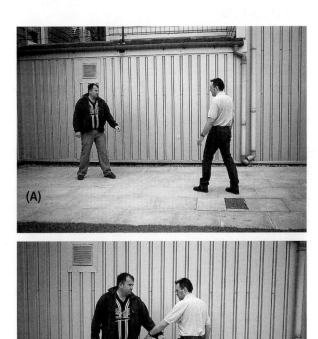

**Figure 8.1** (A) Aggressor (on left) squares up to practitioner who maintains
his distance. (B) Aggressor closes distance in order to press the advantage
(practitioners may elect to close the distance themselves if they feel the need
to take control of the situation). Practitioner begins to position his arm, ready
to apply a control if necessary.

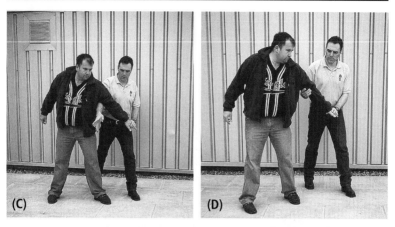

**Figure 8.1** (C) Practitioner takes hold of the aggressor's leading wrist, whilst stepping to the outside of the aggressors arm to establish safe control. (D) By taking firmly hold of the aggressor's arm just above the elbow it is now possible for the practitioner to escort the subject safely, provided there is not too great a difference in size, weight or strength.

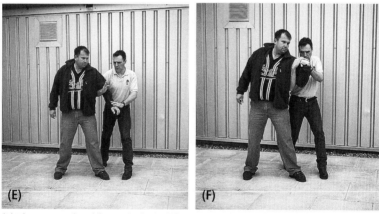

(E) The move should conclude at (D). However, should the aggressor begin to struggle or should there be too great a difference in size, weight or strength, practitioners can progress the technique by pulling the escorting hand firmly into the inside of the elbow joint, enabling control to ... (F) ... apply a swan-neck wrist lock, which permits a greater degree of control or safety. The swan-neck lock is a simple, secure progression of the initial technique, although it must always be applied *with care* and only when no other control method is available.

### Medical implications

The arm control technique is very low risk, but the swan-neck wrist lock carries risk of injury to wrists, through fractures or simple sprains, particularly if subjects resist strongly, necessitating the application of more pressure. The swan-neck technique therefore is medium- to high-risk, depending on level of resistance. Practitioners need to be aware that pain-inducing control techniques applied to joints will always carry a high risk of potential damage, particularly if subjects are experiencing acute behavioural disturbances and/or have an increased pain threshold.

The technique illustrated in Figure 8.1 begins with both exponents facing one another. It will work for any other scenario and would, in fact, be easier to apply from the side or behind. It is far more efficient and safer for two practitioners to apply the technique together, with a third person possibly working as a cover. For safety it is also recommended that practitioners tuck the head in behind subjects' shoulders (see Figure 8.1(E)) to limit the risk of them being struck with the free hand.

The 'swan-neck' type of transport wrist lock should always be used in teams and is not ideally suited to single-practitioner application. However, in some instances, where support is not available, it may be applied successfully, provided there is not too great a size and strength difference between practitioners and clients.

## GOOD AND BAD CONTROLLING TECHNIQUE

Whilst confronting an aggressive client alone is bad practice, in extreme situations it may be necessary. Ideally, sooner than approach alone, practitioners should withdraw. With a duty of care to clients, and consideration for the safety of others in the vicinity, it may become necessary – although never recommended or advised – to attempt a solo control technique. In such circumstances good control is of the utmost importance to avoid further escalation of the situation (Figure 8.2 and Figure 8.3).

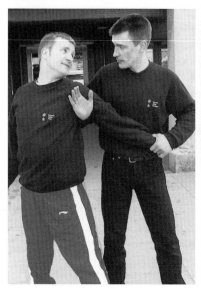

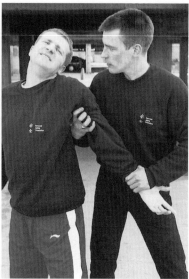

**Figure 8.2** Good – practitioner tucked close behind, using his body to limit the aggressor and allow for communication without any pain.

**Figure 8.3** Bad – practitioner is gripping aggressor's upper arm tightly, causing discomfort or even pain. This could lead to an increase in aggression, and may also inflict bruising.

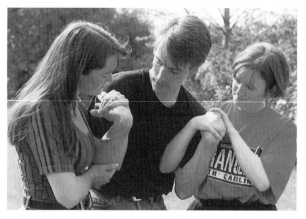

**Figure 8.4** Traditional control and restraint techniques such as the 'swan-neck' wrist lock should only ever be used in extreme situations and with considerable caution. Ideally applied in teams, even using a third practitioner to restrict subjects' head movement, the injury potential is reduced even further.

## PROGRESSION TECHNIQUE FOR INCREASED

## SAFE CONTROL

This technique is a progression of the simple escort control outlined in Figures 8.2 to 8.4, but allows for a greater degree of control and therefore an increased level of safety for service-providers. It is *not* ratified for clinical application and carries with it a high risk potential for injury. Therefore, it is only ever to be considered as a last resort, to be applied by a lone individual who is unable to facilitate an escape and is under threat of severe personal danger from a subject. Equally, the technique could be used to control subjects who may pose a severe risk to others. It is more suited for security personnel than clinical practitioner applications, but if learnt properly has potential for either application under the right, justifiable, circumstances.

### Medical Implications

High risk. If the technique is applied with excess force, or if subjects struggle strongly or are weak, there is a risk of potential damage to shoulders, elbow joints or wrist.

As already outlined, control-type techniques should only ever be used by qualified, experienced practitioners, and then only with extreme caution and consideration to clients. Reckless use or application by unqualified or inexperienced personnel will introduce a high risk factor for injury either to clients or staff.

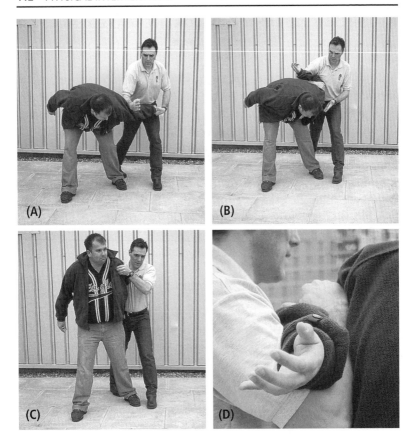

**Figure 8.5** (A) Following on from Figure 8.4, the practitioner (on right) applies a forward arm bar to the aggressor's upper arm (*not to the elbow*) in order to break his balance and allow further access and control of the arm. (B) The practitioner then feeds the aggressor's controlled arm over the top of his closest arm, which had applied the arm bar, and pushes upwards with the elbow and downwards with the wrist. (C) Using his free hand the practitioner pulls the aggressor upright with pressure into the shoulder, whilst still maintaining controlling pressure onto the arm. (D) Close-up of finish position (C) from the rear angle.

## Chapter 9

# UNDERSTANDING AND MANAGING DIVERSE BEHAVIOURS

## INTRODUCTION

The purpose of this book is to introduce the reader to the subject of managing violence and aggression. In order to manage the majority of potential scenarios effectively it may be necessary to understand certain behaviours.

Human behaviour has been studied for many years, from many angles and for many different reasons. Humans, as a society, have a set of values which dictate how we should, or should not, act in any given situation or environment. This is what is seen as 'normal' behaviour.

To understand what is seen to be 'normal' behaviour, first of all, we must understand behaviour as a term or definition. A behaviour is anything that may be 'seen or measured'.

Individuals act and function within the parameters of society and its boundaries most of the time, some more, some less than others. The reasons for deviation from the 'norm' are many, for example hardship, stress, greed or anger to name a few. However, such deviation usually has a reason for it, even if individuals themselves are not aware of it. This is why it is important to reiterate awareness (p. 23) and positive attitudes (p. 27) so that we can begin to recognize, understand and attempt to manage diverse behaviours.

Almost any violent or aggressive act will be considered diverse. They can be measured as such against what society dictates as normal and acceptable. There are different strategies for managing aggressive behaviour effectively.

# PROACTIVE VERSUS REACTIVE STRATEGIES

Why is the emphasis on minimum physical intervention often misconstrued to the point of taking unnecessary risks? The results of an independent Personal Safety Promotion (PSP) survey in 1997 established that 89 per cent of care workers did not know how they could or could not react, given a predictable violent episode. Those surveyed were 'in service' and attending refresher courses for the management of aggression and breakaway training. Although the courses were designed as refreshers, more than 60 per cent of those questioned had never previously received any training. Many understood certain legal boundaries, but could not rationalize or reiterate any set guidelines.

Reactive intervention is usually the response to a challenging situation. In practice this is usually being seen to cope, whilst acting in a professional manner and adhering to policy and procedure. The policy and procedure themselves are often laid down roughly, giving rise to 'grey' areas.

Reactive intervention need not give rise to emergency strategies when given a little forethought and planning. This may seem a contradiction in terms but in practice can work extremely well.

Proactive strategies, planned well, documented and validated, and ratified by the management of an organization, are by far the best plans to ensure success. But there is room for a proactive/reactive strategy.

To be reactive in a situation involves the element of surprise, usually unco-ordinated and unpredictable, allowing a margin for error and for accidents or mistakes. This approach may be fine-tuned to minimize risk to an acceptable and safe level. All that is needed is common sense, control and an ability to rationalize one's own belief system.

An example: a client (or even a stranger) approaches you, spits in your face and then casually walks away. Your reaction could be either (1) any of – anger, resentment, upset or fear – leading to a reactive mechanism response: *loss of control;* or (2) composure (with anger/upset minimized) leading to proactive mechanism: *control of feelings.*

Control does not necessarily mean 'power', it means having control of your own reactions, emotions and dignity. The above example may be seen as extreme but it is a realistic and possible scenario in some fields of care. Should response (1) occur then the situation could very easily escalate into an unmanageable physical confrontation. Option (2) leaves you in control with dignity, enables the situation to be rationalized and will assist in avoiding any potential escalation.

Aggressive subjects will probably be expecting an aggressive response. The lack of such a return can have a positive result, giving them time to rationalize their own feelings or actions. Reacting to a situation with anger, resentment, upset or fear will result in spontaneous responses only: probably negative. To act with composure and confidence is a lot harder to do, but will invariably enable you to manage situations with skill.

Being aware of the possibility of different assaults will not necessarily preclude them from occurring but will enable you to consider an appropriate response. Simply, to formulate a proactive/reactive strategy (see Table 9.1).

**Table 9.1** Maintaining control – guidelines

| Do | Don't |
| --- | --- |
| Adopt a calm and non-threatening stance | Argue or respond to an individual's behaviour in a negative manner |
| Other team members should observe only discreetly | Go in 'mob-handed' |
| Ignore threats or verbal abuse | Challenge or retort to the person |
| Offer reassurance and explanations as to what is happening and why | Shout or show anger or resentment of the incident |
| If you feel you may be making the situation worse, withdraw and allow someone else to negotiate | Adopt a confrontational stance |
| Adhere strictly to guidelines, codes of conduct and planned intervention strategies | Try to bend the rules or to 're-invent the wheel' |
| Only use the minimum required force for the shortest possible time to control any physical intervention | Never slap, punch or kick the individual without justification and try not to use inappropriate holds or locks |

# Chapter 10

# POST-INCIDENT

## INTRODUCTION

After any form of physical or verbal confrontation all those involved will experience various emotions, which can include being depressed, elated, helpless, scared or worried. In addition to this they will also probably still have an excess of adrenalin coursing through them and may be unsettled and anxious. Depending on the individuals concerned, or the severity of the incident, they may experience an emotional imbalance for a long period after the event. In severe instances some individuals may never fully recover.

It is easy to look back and feel that a situation could have been managed more effectively and state how this might be done, but this is a more useful exercise when considering the future. It means learning by experience. What about the individuals directly involved in the incident? How might they feel? What will be their future opinions and feelings if a similar incident where to happen again?

Any trauma, no matter how minor, will give rise to some form of stress, whether it be behavioural or emotional. It will have some effect on individuals' psychological stability. In behavioural terms, whatever happens as a direct result of an experience will reinforce the natural reaction of individuals if they were to have the same or similar experience again.

It is important for individuals to be able to rationalize their own feelings and thoughts on a given situation that they may have experienced. It is also important for them to learn positive coping mechanisms, not only for everyday stresses but also for traumatic life events. It is therefore useful to have some means of informal counselling or debriefing after traumatic incidents.

# AFTER THE EVENT

There is growing recognition of the need for effective management of situations after the event, yet many employers, including major organizations, are unaware of the importance of a post-incident policy. Although managers may have heard of post-traumatic stress disorder (PTSD), often they cannot identify it or relate to it. Good management is always considered to be proactive, but there also has to be flexibility to permit good reactive management should circumstances dictate this.

Although not everyone who experiences a violent episode will be affected seriously or in the long term, others find it difficult to rationalize such incidents and their subsequent emotions will affect their work and relationships with others. A common result may be feelings of vulnerability and fear of other such episodes occurring. This can lead to individuals giving up work or being unable to work properly. They may also decide to take up self-defence sessions to ensure that the same thing does not happen again. PSP has found, somewhat ironically, that most of the companies or individuals that book self-defence and personal safety courses do so as the result of incidents that have already happened.

Those people who manage episodes better are generally those who have encountered such incidents previously or those who have attended specialist training for their vocation that included the management of violence and aggression. Knowing that they may have to deal with violence and aggression in their work or everyday life will equip people better to deal with it and will also allow them to rationalize it more easily should it happen. If service-providers have no idea that they might encounter violent situations, particularly in the workplace, they will have difficulty in quantifying such episodes and post-incident their emotions will be amplified. It is better to inform all prospective employees of the potential risks and let them make a conscious decision as to whether to pursue that vocation than to let them find out when it is too late and they have to suffer the consequences.

After any violent episode it is important that all those concerned are debriefed. Debriefing is not necessarily an investigation and need not be undertaken by a senior member of staff, although in most situations it will be deemed a management responsibility. Other than finding out the facts of an incident in order to implement strategies to avoid other such occurrences in the future, the main purpose of debriefing must be to help victims to tell somebody about the episode. Those involved will invariably want to talk to somebody about the event but, more importantly, whether they feel they want to talk or not, they will need to. This will enable them to rationalize the event and the part they played in it.

## DEBRIEFING

Debriefing is not an inquest. Individuals concerned will need reassurance and possibly comfort. It is not an issue of 'tea and sympathy', but more an opportunity for them to express their feelings and concerns regarding the episode and for a listener to reassure them, whilst being entirely honest and open. Debriefing is best undertaken by individuals with counselling experience and requires the simple skill of being able to listen. Empathy is vital, but not sympathy, and tactics such as personal disclosure (see p. 48) may prove extremely beneficial. This may entail counsellors divulging a relevant story of a similar incident in which they may have been involved, using it to lessen the isolation or any feelings of inadequecy that individuals may be suffering.

A mistake often made by employers is to send individuals involved home after an incident or to tell them to take some time off. Unless there is physical injury that necessitates it this is not always the best solution and may result in individuals sitting at home alone worrying about an incident and allowing their emotions to take control of them. Continuing to work alongside their friends and colleagues can, in many cases, give a sense of normality and provides a focus point away from the incident. Individuals may still need some form of counselling, otherwise they could just try and avoid the issue without ever having actually addressed or rationalized it. In more serious cases, individuals will be unable to face work or their friends and will normally require professional counselling beyond that available internally through an organization.

## THE 'EMOTIONAL BALANCE'

People always have a 'normal' emotional balance, which is where they will have been before an incident. As a confrontation occurs there is a steep rise in emotions – as adrenalin and noradrenalin are released (see p. 34) – ultimately reaching a peak at which they are most involved. Once the incident has passed, there is a 'fall-off' of emotions, at varying rates for different people, much as the peak reached will vary from person to person. The important point is that when the emotional rate drops it generally falls below the 'normal' balance, and can often stay below that level for a long period, depending on how affected by the incident individuals may be.

It could be potentially dangerous to attempt debriefing while individuals are at an emotional peak, as they are likely to be very emotional, even aggressive, and may well fail to reason clearly. Although there may be value in trying to diffuse an aggressive situation at its peak verbally, this is not considered to be debriefing. Similarly, it is not recommended to attempt debriefing while subjects are on the initial downward emotional curve after an event, as they may still not be in control and need time to regain their composure and reasoning.

The downward emotional curve will continue below the 'normal' baseline, reaching a low point. At this low point, individuals will not be able to rationalize an incident and any attempt to do this could result in a higher state of arousal, exceeding the high emotional level reached at the original peak. When subjects return from the low point to normality, they will be able to discuss an incident rationally with less risk of becoming aroused again. At this level, composure is regained and debriefing is of the most value to both aggressors and diffusers.

The exception to this occurs when individuals reach the nadir, below the initial emotional balance before an incident, but then fail to recover that normal level. In this instance they should be referred for specialist counselling.

After any incident, regardless of whether those involved demonstrate any outward signs of having been affected, debriefing is of the utmost importance. Debriefing should only be facilitated by appropriately qualified individuals, with the relevant skills and experience, such as a counsellor or senior personnel manager, although any member of staff may have the skills required. If it is felt that there is nobody appropriate within the establishment, the individuals concerned should be referred to an external consultant.

## Case study

*Background*

Amy is a 32-year-old care assistant, working towards her National Vocational Qualification at level three in direct care. She started her career working with elderly, mentally ill patients, and then chose to work with clients of a younger generation who had more complex needs. Their needs are those of a small population of society who, realistically, will always require a level of support that means their lives will always have input from others, that is, carers, doctors or social workers.

*Fact*

There is an emphasis on individual care, always taking an holistic approach. However, because of the needs presented there is an element of a secure environment.

During the five years that Amy has worked with this group of people, she has been seriously assaulted on three occasions by a client, ultimately resulting in her being transferred to a less stressful environment, without choice, and with very little support.

As every manager will acknowledge, sometimes it is better to relocate a member of staff to solve an immediate problem. However, in the long term, how many staff can you relocate without addressing the core issue? It is often easier to brush things aside than to deal with the problem in hand.

Amy incurred six sutures in her left cheek as a result of being attacked with a piece of plastic fashioned as a weapon from a wristwatch. The management decision, after a period of convalescence, was to move Amy to a less stressful environment with no counselling or support.

*To date*

At the time of publishing, Amy is working in a new environment, as a competent and professional carer, having almost finished her studies. She has a permanent scar to her left cheek and has not been paid for her time 'off sick', as her employers do not count the incident as serious enough for this. She could prosecute personally; however, in her own words, *'It's not his fault, it is not worth the trauma . . .'*

## CONCLUSION

Careful management of the environment and structuring of the work team could possibly have helped Amy to avoid being exposed to a potential risk in the first instance, but this is not always possible and, even with the best management, incidents will still occur. A high degree of training, supported by practice and refresher training could possibly have assisted Amy to avoid becoming injured, although, again, this is not always realistic. An increased sense of awareness would also contribute to safety, but even then the risk potential can never be erased. All the principles outlined throughout this book could contribute positively to avoiding such incidents, or to lessen the risk of them happening.

The one thing that is not a variable, that may be assured, is that if an incident does occur, those involved will need some form of post-incident debriefing and counselling. Different individuals may require differing degrees of input, but all will require some. Beyond counselling, additional support should be made available to reintegrate individuals back into their roles.

# Chapter 11

# EXTERNAL RISK MANAGEMENT AND PERSONAL SAFETY

## INTRODUCTION

Although assaults within the workplace are a major concern, it should also be realized that many incidents also occur while attending, or travelling to or from, home visits or other associated centres.

Attacks outside the establishment often have completely different motives. Incidents in the workplace may be fuelled by numerous factors, which are generally related to the type of establishment or the policy therein, but can be managed or prepared for. The motives for external attacks are often more basic, but can also be managed by combining basic knowledge of personal safety with an increased degree of awareness.

Effective personal safety involves individuals managing themselves proactively. Understanding the motives and methods of aggressors will enable them to implement simple strategies to reduce their risk of becoming potential targets.

However, certain motives remain unchanged. If clients are suffering pain, frustration or confusion while they are being treated during a home visit, it is possible that they may become aggressive. Similarly, their families or associates may become hostile if the treatment they witness does not meet expectations.

There is also the risk of falling victim to more readily identified external motives, such as theft. Thieves may perceive a bag to be of some significant value and have no hesitation in using violence in order to obtain it. Equally, vehicles such as ambulances may readily be identified as carrying expensive equipment or drugs.

All of us need to be aware of the risk of street crime – a problem that, despite advances in policing, continues to plague society. The head of the London Metropolitan Police, Sir John Stevens, addressed students at the University of Leicester in March 2002, confessing, 'We see robbers with strings of convictions, strutting across the estates of inner London, having won their most recent game in court – arrogant, untouchable, fearless and ready for anything.' Highlighting the honesty of the Commissioner, the Daily Mirror outlined his conclusions, 'It is not uncommon to have muggers released on bail eight or nine times before they face trial. The level of violence we are witnessing by robbers intent on stealing is quite unprecedented.'[19]

The majority of perpetrators of street crime will have at least a basic plan of what they intend to do. Such a plan may be as simple as establishing an opportune location for the crime and an easy escape route, but this still constitutes a simplistic form of plan. Victims, however, usually do not have a plan at all, primarily because they do not know they are going to become victims. This is the one single reason why numerous street offenders are successful. They take their victims by surprise, having a basic plan or pattern for their assault, as opposed to their intended targets, who do not.

Regardless of the motive for the attack, the main priority for victims must be to escape as soon as they can, immediately if possible. The longer they spend with an attacker the greater the risk of their being seriously injured, or worse. Standing and fighting should never be considered as an option because victims do not know the potential or desperation of aggressors, or whether they have accomplices or are armed with an undisclosed weapon. The priority of escape is the first, and most important, strategy to be remembered.

When considering personal safety it is always wise to remember that avoidance is always better than cure, and there are various guidelines and strategies that may be used to promote personal safety when working in the field.

## JOURNEY PLANNING

When travelling, a basic journey plan is a simple means of ensuring consideration is given to factors such as destination, mode of transport, possible route and time required. Although some organizations insist that personnel use a journey plan for management purposes, the reality is that they can prove invaluable in ensuring safety *en route*.

A simple journey plan consists of making a list of all proposed calls, along with the anticipated calling times and expected duration or purpose of the call (Table 11.1). A simple plan can take less than five minutes to formulate and when completed a copy can be left with colleagues so that relevant steps may be taken should there be any cause for concern, such as late return or a failure to arrive. Form the habit of calling either the office or home if ever running late as this will support the journey plan and allay any fears. With this habit established, any failure to call home would again indicate a potential problem.

**Table 11.1** Example of a basic journey plan

| Time | Location/client | Reason for call | Contact no. |
|------|-----------------|-----------------|-------------|
| 0930 | Office | Collect bag | 0151 727 0000 |
| 1030 | Mrs Smith 45 Parkway Road | Home visit | Mobile |
| 1130 | Ms Jones 100 Victory Close | Home visit | Mobile or 0151 727 0001 |

The most important aspect of a journey plan is that it makes people think about exactly where they are going, including when they are going and the route they are thinking of taking. A call that requires travelling into an unknown rural area after dark, for example, might be rescheduled to help avoid any compromise in potential safety.

Society often defines good and bad areas by social class and wealth. Some people will instinctively try to avoid 'bad' areas because of fear for their safety or of crime. Although there may be some truth in these perceptions these so-called 'bad' areas still need to be serviced and the residents still have a right to care.

If a practitioner has eight calls to make in one day then timing becomes an important factor. Any potential risk areas should ideally be visited first thing in the morning, before the community is fully awake, but preferably in daylight. Calling in such areas during the dark increases the risk factor. It would also be unwise to embark on a trip at night along secluded lanes or in a region that is unfamiliar, particularly if the same journey could be rescheduled into daylight hours. Planning can also extend to plotting a safe course to avoid 'bad' areas or isolated regions.

The problems of large housing projects and inner city estates are frequently documented, but most crime is usually committed by a small hardcore of individuals. These offenders will loiter, sometimes out of sight, in anticipation of unknowing people who may stray into their territory. Strangers can usually be easily identified and are ideal targets for opportunist crimes, such as vehicle and property theft. Other residents within a depressed community are not normally the main targets as they often do not have a great deal worth stealing but, more significantly, could possibly identify the perpetrators.

## SAFETY ON FOOT

Anybody walking alone is instantly vulnerable. By remaining aware and taking simple precautions the risk of being attacked may be greatly reduced.

When on foot journey planning becomes even more important, although it is more likely to take the form of careful consideration as opposed to actual documentation. Short-cuts through alleyways, underpasses or across parks and waste ground should be avoided. These are commonly termed 'black spots' because of their secluded or isolated nature, providing ideal locations for potential assailants to lie in wait. It is far better for individuals to add a little time to their journey and ensure safe arrival than to risk a potentially dangerous short-cut. This is also true regardless of the weather conditions. Taking an ill-advised short-cut to limit exposure to bad weather would not necessarily limit the risk factor.

When walking on the pavement it is good practice to face oncoming traffic, making it more difficult for a car to pull up from behind unnoticed. Walking near the kerb of the pavement will make it harder for attackers to reach potential victims from a driveway or alley. However, it would not be advisable to walk right on the edge of the pavement as this leaves individuals vulnerable to being accosted from a passing or parked vehicle (Figure 11.1).

If there is a reason for someone to believe that they are being followed then a good strategy is to cross the road in order to see if the suspect follows. Should they do so then crossing back will confirm ultimately whether it is coincidence or mere paranoia. Having established that someone may be following you it is important to get to a busy public place, such as a public house, and telephone the police. Telephone boxes should be avoided as it is possible to become trapped inside them. Such instances validate further the use of mobile telephones.

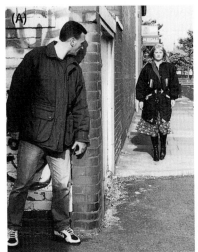
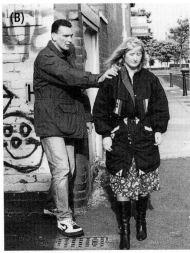
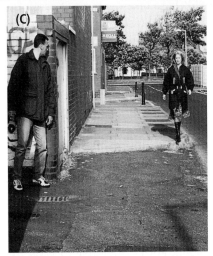

**Figure 11.1** Avoid 'black spots' such as alleyways. (A) No: when walking on the pavement walk kerbside. (B) Walking close to a wall or hedgerow makes you an easy target. (C) Yes: by walking kerbside it makes it difficult for a potential attacker to reach you.

Wearing expensive clothes and jewellery can instantly identify somebody as a target, as can showing expensive mobile telephones. For those who do not wear a uniform for work it is wise to consider where exactly they are going and to then dress accordingly. In any physical encounter clothes may be torn or otherwise damaged –

again supporting the idea of considering what attire is appropriate to the work being undertaken.

Keys and forms of identity should ideally not be carried together in the same bag or pocket. Similarly, cheque books, credit cards and bank correspondence could also be kept in separate locations, such as jacket pockets. Thieves will rarely wait around to get every single item from every pocket and consequently certain items can be rendered valueless if accompanying matter is not also acquired. House keys are no good without an address and the value of a cheque book automatically decreases without an appropriate card or pattern signature.

## SAFETY IN THE CAR

Journey planning once again becomes of paramount importance when travelling by car. Many individuals set off on journeys without actually knowing the precise location of their destination, or indeed exactly how they are going to get there. It is not uncommon for people to find themselves many miles away from home in completely unfamiliar surroundings.

Regardless of location, it is good practice to stay in the car as much as possible and to keep the doors locked and the windows closed. Should practitioners be involved in a traffic accident the emergency services are more than capable of opening any vehicle, whether or not the doors are locked. The crime of 'car-jacking' is becoming more and more prevalent and involves a vehicle, often including its occupants, being hijacked whilst stationary at traffic lights or a road junction. With increasingly advanced car security systems in place this is now proving a far easier way for thieves to procure cars.

Bags and personal possessions, particularly valuables, should never be left unattended in a car. If they cannot be removed, or it is impractical to remove them, they should be locked out of sight in the boot or glovebox. A car is an easy target for an opportunist, who can break in and steal a bag within seconds, regardless of whether there is anybody actually in the vehicle.

People can take on a totally different personality when in the assumed safety of their own vehicles. 'Road rage' has become a commonly acknowledged problem, which has the potential to escalate into a severe confrontation. The temptation to respond to other drivers with verbal abuse or hand gestures is unnecessary and should always be resisted as it can rapidly progress into a more serious incident.

Although home visits cannot always be scheduled for the benefit of practitioners, it is wise for drivers to take into consideration what time of day they will be returning to their vehicles (Figure 11.2A). If parking in a busy, well-lit street or multi-storey car park during daylight, consideration should be given as to how that location may change after dark. The same street or car park can radically change at night into a dimly lit 'black spot'. On returning to a vehicle it is advisable to have the keys ready and to quickly check around the car, if only to confirm that it still has four wheels. The interior of the car should also be subject to a quick check, particularly the back seat, before getting in. A small torch is a useful item to carry for such purposes, some of which are found in key fobs.

If practitioners are using their own vehicles for work, membership of a reputable breakdown service is a wise precaution, although regular servicing and proper maintenance will reduce the chances of a car leaving them stranded. It should not be assumed that recovery membership means car maintenance can be compromised. Depending on workload, a recovery service may take more than an hour to reach a stranded motorist (Figure 11.2B).

Regular checks of oil and water levels should become second nature, as should checking tyre pressures and treads, including the spare wheel. Standard safety items that should be found in every car are a basic tool kit, a jack and jack handle, first aid kit, warning triangle and spare fuel in an approved safety container. Various minor breakdowns could potentially be repaired by drivers themselves if they have the correct items. A warning light is an indicator of a potential problem and therefore should never be ignored. A more basic consideration is to ensure that there are appropriate funds or credit facilities to keep the vehicle fuelled during the journey.

Part of the journey planning process also includes looking at the weather and taking any appropriate precautions. Snow, heavy rain, strong winds and severe fog can all leave drivers stranded. Traffic reports and up-to-date maps will also figure in the preparations, helping to avoid delays and possible unknown detours.

If working in rural areas it is prudent to take note of payphones, service stations and public houses as they are passed. In the instance of a breakdown it may prove better to walk back to a known telephone than to walk ahead in the hope of finding one. The necessity of having a mobile telephone is further supported when considering the potential risks of covering any large area for work calls or home visits.

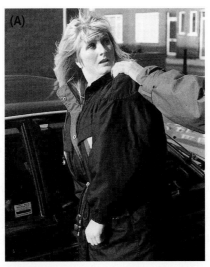

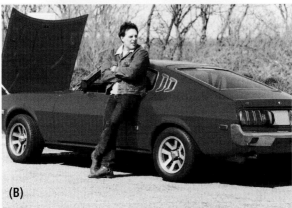

**Figure 11.2** (A) When parking a vehicle the safety of the surrounding area requires due consideration. (B) Regular maintenance will help ensure that a car does not leave the practitioner stranded in a potentially vulnerable location.

## PUBLIC TRANSPORT

Many people, including practitioners, use public transport, either out of convenience, cost or simply through not having access to a personal vehicle. Although most public transport is perfectly safe there are still some precautions that require consideration.

When using buses, isolated bus stops should be avoided if at all possible, particularly after dark. If travelling on an empty bus it is prudent to sit near to the driver or if travelling by rail, close to the driver or guard's compartment. Empty train carriages should also be avoided and on embarkation pay attention to where the communication cord is located. If a confrontation should occur and no assistance can be summoned from other passengers there is a justifiable case for using a communication cord. Selecting a train carriage that will stop close to the exit at the destination station will negate any extended walking along potentially dark platforms.

If ordering a taxi it is wise to always use a reputable firm and, if possible, book by telephone or directly at a taxi office. Although black cabs can be hailed, it is illegal for minicabs to stop when flagged down. Check that the taxi that arrives is actually the one that was ordered. Asking for a description of the car, colour, make, etc., will assist in this, but also it should be noted that all taxis must be plated and show clearly driver details and numbers.

When using a taxi it is good practice to sit behind the driver and never to divulge any personal details to them. If there is any reason for concern the driver should be told to pull over at the nearest well-lit public area and the passenger should immediately get out. If there is any doubt whatsoever, the car should be avoided and an alternative considered.

## SAFETY IN THE HOME

Safety at home is not necessarily a consideration for clinical practitioners, and how it would affect their working practice is open to debate unless they worked primarily from home, but personal safety and well-being should always be accepted as a relevant issue, regardless of location or profession.

To ensure safety at home it is recommended that the property is well-secured, with strong locks and possibly even an alarm, ideally with a panic button facility. Keys should always be readily accessible in the instance of fire or of having to vacate the property to avoid an intruder. Anybody moving into a new property should change the locks immediately, to eliminate any problems from individuals who may be holding old keys.

Only initials and a surname should be used in telephone listings or on doorplates, making it difficult for strangers to establish whether a man or a woman is in residence. When answering the telephone a simple 'Hello' will not divulge more information than is necessary. In the instance of a wrong number it is better to ask the caller to repeat the number they want, sooner than revealing any personal information. In the instance of abusive or threatening telephone calls a good response is to place the receiver down beside the telephone and to walk away. Returning a few minutes later and replacing the receiver will deny the caller any satisfaction from getting a response. If such calls were to persist they need to be reported to the police and to the telephone company.

If selling a property it is advisable not to show people around unaccompanied as this could leave vendors potentially vulnerable. Equally, returning home alone at night to a property can leave residents exposed and so the use of movement-sensitive lighting is invaluable. Should there be signs of a break-in it should not be considered safe to enter the property until the police have been in attendance and declared it clear.

Drawing the curtains after dark will deter prowlers and caution should always be exercised when answering the door. The use of a strong chain, intercom or door-mounted 'spy hole' will assist in establishing the identity of any unannounced visitors.

## PERSONAL ALARMS

If involved in an aggressive confrontation in a public location there is a great benefit in using noise to create a scene or to possibly summon assistance. Should a situation become violent shouting, 'Get off!' loudly and repeatedly will draw attention to the situation, causing potential embarrassment to the aggressor and also highlighting to them instantly that there are witnesses around them.

There are, however, limitations to shouting and committed or confused assailants may not cease their activity. Equally, victims may be unable to shout, possibly through fear, or transgressors may try to shut them up. Personal attack alarms provide a logical and very effective alternative.

There is a comprehensive range of personal alarms available, ranging from gas-filled screech alarms to electronic devices, some of which incorporate motion alarms and integral torches. The majority of alarms are relatively cheap and extremely effective. Designed to fit into the palm of the hand, when activated they emit a loud screech, often more than 120 decibels in volume, which works to help deter any aggressor and possibly to summon assistance (Figure 11.3).

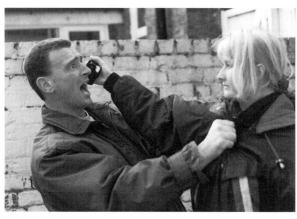

**Figure 11.3** Personal alarms can prove vital if working out in the community.

The reason for the validity of such alarms is that most assailants will pick on what they consider to be relatively easy targets, and hope to avoid a protracted skirmish or one they may not be able to win. They may well also have planned their attack to some degree. Consequently, they will feel that they have some control of the situation. A screeching alarm suddenly takes that element of control away from them, primarily because it did not figure in the original plan. Not wanting to get caught, as well as no longer being in control, and with their strategy, however basic, crumbling, the most obvious course of action is to withdraw.

Aggressors who launch a spontaneous attack, or who have simply just lost control, will be instantly snapped back to reality by the sound of an alarm.

The case for such alarms is further strengthened by the fact that, on a fresh battery, an electronic alarm is capable of sounding for more than two hours. Most are activated by the sharp removal of a hand grenade-style pin. Should the intended victim remove the pin and throw it away an assailant is unlikely to try and retrieve it. To silence the alarm an aggressor would have to prise it from the defender's grasp, throw it on to the ground and then stamp on it, possibly repeatedly.

Any noise can prove a good deterrent and therefore people may consider screaming or shouting loudly as an alternative to an alarm. In an extreme threat situation, however, due to fear or panic victims can sometimes find they are unable to scream. Should they be able to do so then the attacker could panic and will probably take one of two courses of action. The first is to withdraw, whereas the second would be to try and silence the target. Assailants may not easily be able to cover the victim's mouth with their hands, but may find it simpler to punch, strike or choke their subjects into silence. They can punch somebody as often, or as hard, as they like but it will not silence an alarm.

It is not unheard of for people to have alarms and then proceed to leave them at home. An alarm at home is no good to them. Before venturing out, alarms should be tested to ensure that they work correctly. An alarm with a flat battery is of no use to anybody. Anyone carrying an alarm should have it readily to hand, ideally on a bag strap or belt clip, possibly even in the palm of the hand. An alarm at the bottom of a bag is of no use, particularly if the bag is stolen.

An alarm is a good comforter. Merely knowing that they have an alarm, something that can be called upon in a difficult situation, is very reassuring for some people. Alarms can easily be carried in the workplace, the street or when travelling by almost any mode of transport. If individuals have personal alarms they could save their lives. If they do not have alarms they cannot save them.

It may be tempting to carry some form of other personal safety device but that should never be considered as an option. Carrying anything that may be considered a weapon is totally unethical and potentially leaves individuals liable to prosecution. A further consideration is that for a weapon, even an everyday item employed as an incidental weapon, to be of any real use the bearer must be able to use it effectively. If they are not proficient in its use then it could possibly be taken from them and used against them.

## SAFETY IN THE DEPARTMENT OR ON THE WARD

In any secure unit, good-quality door and window locks are essential to maintain control within the building. Panic buttons linked to a central alarm system are usually placed strategically throughout the building and may be activated should a situation become unmanageable. These concepts can readily be adopted on any ward or unit, secure or otherwise.

On a secure unit the most likely risk of attack comes from clients themselves, but on a general ward there is a risk of assault from the general public, including clients, their relatives or associates. Intruders may also wander into the department in search of drugs or other items of value. These individuals, too, can create problems if approached. It is the employers' responsibility to ensure a safe working environment for employees. Under Section 2 (1) of the Health and Safety at Work Act 1974, employers must ensure, so far as is reasonable, the health, safety and welfare at work of their employees. This would also include taking appropriate and reasonable steps to protect them from assault.

Three main causative factors for employees to be attacked in the workplace by a member of the public are either lack of information, lack of service or the actual environment itself (see p. 8). These factors also apply to clinical environments, particularly within areas such as casualty departments.

All three causative factors may be managed correctly by employers and it is their responsibility to try to do so. Service will always be a difficult issue to address, due primarily to workload and restrictions of time and personnel, but provided the highest level possible is striven for, and clients and their associates are kept appraised, it may be controlled to some degree. Communication is of the utmost importance, particularly if protracted waiting times are anticipated.

Catalysts (see p. 14), such as alcohol and drugs, can play a major part in fuelling violence within casualty departments. Public waiting areas can be monitored by CCTV and the use of security staff should ensure a rapid response to any severe problems. In staff areas, or on private or secure wards, staff identification cards, combined with secure swipe card-activated locks can assist in maintaining the necessary level of security.

Staff may also fall victim to attack from other employees. If any such hostile intent is identified, or indeed, an assault committed, it should be reported immediately to the appropriate line manager. In the instance of a physical assault this can also be reported to the police. Similarly, if a threat is continued outside the workplace, again, it becomes a police matter, although the management of the organization still has some duty to address the issue.

With regard to personal safety, there are countless strategies and ideas that may be employed to avoid confrontations, but most individuals simply do not take the time required to do so. It only takes a few moments to consider a journey plan and to check and stow a personal alarm. It may take slightly longer to walk around the block than it would to take the short-cut through the dark alleyway, but taking those few seconds can make the difference between becoming a victim or not.

Effective personal safety may be likened to a game of percentages. The actual odds of being severely attacked are relatively low, but by employing simple safety strategies they can be reduced even further. By adopting a positive posture, utilizing confident body language and good composure, the odds of being selected as a victim lessen. Being constantly aware, and giving appropriate consideration to surroundings, will also help to decrease the odds. Carrying a personal alarm can give a distinct advantage in a difficult situation and consequently the odds of becoming a victim are reduced even further. Lastly, acquiring a basic knowledge of breakaway techniques, and possibly even self-defence, will provide another significant edge that further reduces the odds of becoming a victim.

# CONCLUSION

This handbook has been structured solely to provide an introductory insight to the issue of managing violence and aggression, with the emphasis strongly on personal safety and the validity of breakaway techniques. It is not, however, intended to be a comprehensive guide, and therefore further research into the subject would always be recommended, particularly for clinical practitioners working directly with clients.

The connection between aggression and the health care services has been explored throughout the text, although it can be summarized by Mason and Chandley:

> The threat of violence is of concern to all members of society and more so to members of the health care professions, whose task it is to care for those who are in need, but who may also be violent. Those who attack others also tend to be hurt in the process and ultimately are brought into contact with health professional, either in casualty departments or psychiatric services. If the violent person has an accompanying disorder, such as a learning difficulty, mental disorder, personality disorder or drug addiction, then the aggression becomes part of the 'medical problem'.[20]

Personal safety, awareness and avoidance are the primary considerations. It is also hoped that through the work the reader will gain a basic understanding of the principles of breakaway techniques, and their importance.

The practical techniques illustrated are those as taught in hospitals and schools of health studies, for application in a variety of situations. The techniques are all effective and proven in use, but consideration must always be given to the circumstances under which they are to be used, including the nature of aggressors and the relevant impact factors, including the possible consequences of the application, medical and otherwise.

In order to be successful in application the techniques need to be practised regularly and the accompanying text reviewed. In use, the techniques need not be totally accurate or utterly precise, but they must work when applied and the further they are removed from that illustrated, the greater the risk of injury either to practitioners or subjects. The use of techniques must also be ethical and in keeping with policy and procedure applicable to the environment.

This handbook is not intended as a stand-alone learning tool. It is intended as a reference work to accompany a specialist course. Books have obvious limitations and therefore should never be considered as a realistic alternative to attending an actual training course. On completion of the text, the next step is to enrol on a course if one has not already been undertaken.

It is also accepted that practical training courses have limitations, normally dictated by a lack of time. Traditional one-day sessions will never be enough to cover such a complex subject and, consequently, this handbook will provide invaluable supplementary learning and a solid reference to reinforce learning. An ideal format for a practical course would be to run over a period of weekly sessions, each lasting no more than two hours, which would allow for private study and review. This is an important factor to consider when trying either to organize or attend a course.

Specialists in physical intervention techniques include instructors from the police and prison services, but the needs of the clinical profession have dictated that specialist instructors now provide courses aimed solely for that application, generally structured with the purpose of handling challenging behaviours. These specialists have regularly had to use their skills in practice but are likely to have only a limited repertoire of techniques, based upon commonly encountered scenarios, often within controlled or reinforced surroundings. Expert martial artists may well have a far greater depth of knowledge concerning defensive techniques but will be unlikely to understand the principles of 'non-aversive' interventions, or those of ethical restraint. The ideal coach will have extensive experience, knowledge and understanding of both areas.

Whether or not the reader elects to follow this subject further, it is strongly recommended that this book is kept to hand and reviewed periodically. This is particularly important for individuals who operate within the clinical environment, working closely with both clients and the public. It must be understood that physical skills, even simple ones, need constant review and practice to be called upon in an emergency. Similarly, the mind must also be conversant with management principles if situations are to be avoided or managed by any physical response.

The final points for consideration are that all situations can be managed effectively, provided those involved are conversant with the basics. Proper management of the environment, staff and self, combined with a clearly defined and easily understood policy should considerably reduce, or even eliminate, the possibility of violent or aggressive episodes. Competent, well-trained personnel will ensure that if a situation does occur, it will be handled professionally and with minimum fuss.

From the individual practitioner's perspective, regardless of their specific setting, it is apparent that very few receive training at a level, or consistency, that can ensure integrity and enhance professional standards. Returning to the findings of Professor Gournay in the UKCC consultation document, it was highlighted that 'a very large number of respondants had not received any form of training' and that only 'a tiny minority had received refresher training'.[21] These findings were also supported by the feedback provided directly to the PSP training organization by course students, many of whom had been on placement or in service with no training whatsoever.

If training is effective, valuable and needed but seemingly not provided to the standards required, or reviewed to a level to ensure competence, possibly the answer is for practitioners to ensure that they obtain the necessary information, or regularly review themselves any skills they may have been taught. Although this may be politically contentious, and obviously takes possession of an item that organizations or Trusts should be providing for personnel, ultimately, it helps to ensure the personal safety of both practitioners and clients by taking ownership and responsibility. This should not be necessary, but practitioners need to consider that if they are not prepared to make provision for their own safety, they cannot rely on others to do it for them. This work is not necessarily the solution, but it does provide a point from which to start.

# ADDITIONAL INFORMATION

## TRAINING

There are numerous training organizations across the UK that can facilitate courses in non-aversive breakaway or intervention techniques. University schools of health studies can provide links to such organizations, or alternatively, for more details contact PSP, PO Box 127, Southport PR9 7GZ (email: kikentai.uk@btopenworld.com or website: www.p-s-p.com).

# REFERENCES

[1] Coombes, R. Violence – the facts. *Nursing Times*, 28 October 1998, 32. 'Violence – The Facts.'

[2] Department of Health (DoH). NHS set targets to improve quality of working lives for staff. Document 89/390. Wetherby: DoH, 22 September 1998.

[3] Smith, R. Nurse fights for life after car park attack. *Daily Mirror*, 5 February 2000, 4.

[4] Shaw, A. and Fraser, C. Colleagues save doctor after he's knifed in back. *Daily Mirror*, 5 February 2000, 5.

[5] Meikle, J. Rise in attacks on staff 'blighting NHS'. *Guardian*, 29 January 2001, 8.

[6] NHS Health and Development Agency. *Violence and Aggression in General Practice. Guidance on Assessment and Management.* Consultation document, 2001, 4.

[7] Mason, T. and Chandley, M. *Managing Violence and Aggression.* Edinburgh: Churchill Livingstone, 1999, 36.

[8] De Bernieres, L. I was attacked with a bottle, a knife and a baseball bat. *The Times,* 29 March 2001, 2.

[9] Department of Employment. Health & Safety at Work Act, 1974. Statute.

[10] European Convention for Human Rights, 2000. Statute.

[11] Gournay, K. *Recognition, Prevention and Therapeutic Management of Violence in Mental Health Care.* Consultation document. London: United Kingdom Central Council for Nursing, Midwifery and Health Visiting (UKCC), 2001, 18.

[12] Gournay, K. *Recognition, Prevention and Therapeutic Management of Violence in Mental Health Care.* Consultation document. London: UKCC, 2001, 11.

[13] Gournay, K. *Recognition, Prevention and Therapeutic Management of Violence in Mental Health Care*. Consultation document. London: UKCC, 2001, 5.

[14] Morris, N. 300,000 sex attacks a year unreported. *Daily Mirror*, 19 February 2000, 19.

[15] *Collins English Dictionary*. London: William Collins, 1986, 16.

[16] *Collins English Dictionary*. London: William Collins, 1986, 45.

[17] *Collins English Dictionary*. London: William Collins, 1986, 616.

[18] Bilton, T., Bonnet, K., Jones, P., Stanworth, M., Sheard, K. and Webster, A. *Introductory Sociology*. London: Macmillan Educational, 1987, 405.

[19] Hardy, J. Justice system is a joke. *Daily Mirror*, 7 March 2002, 17.

[20] Mason, T. and Chandley, M. *Managing Violence and Aggression*. Edinburgh: Churchill Livingstone, 1999, preface.

[21] Gournay, K. *Recognition, Prevention and Therapeutic Management of Violence in Mental Health Care*. Consultation document. London: UKCC, 2001, 33.

# INDEX

Page numbers in italics refer to figures and tables when separate from related text.

'acute behavioural disturbance' 20
adrenalin 34–5, 38–9, 40, 41
    post-incident 116, 118–19
    *see also* 'fight or flight'
age, as impact factor 32
aggressiveness
    definition 27
    incidence in NHS settings 1–3, 6–7
    *vs* assertiveness 26–9
alarm systems 24
    personal 24, 131–3, 134–5
alcohol 20–1, 32
animated movements, as warning signal 35
appearance
    of confidence 56–7
    influence of 55–6
appropriate clothing 55–6, 77, 126–7
appropriate facial expression 54–5
appropriate responses 30–1, 114–15
arm control techniques 106–9
    good and bad 109, *110*
'The Artful Dodger' 64
assaultive behaviour *30*, *31*
assertiveness
    definition 27
    *vs* aggressiveness 26–9

awareness
    assertiveness *vs* aggressiveness 26–9
    colour code 25–6
    environmental/individual issues 23–5
    knowledge 34, 41–2, 60
    using principles 28–9, 72–3, 74, 113
    warning signals 34–6

'bad' neighbourhoods 124–5
beliefs 21–2, 37, 42
'black' code 26
'black spots' 125, *126*, 128
'bladed' stance 36, *53*
body language 26–7, 28–9, 45, 51–7
    professional approach 53–7
    *see also* communication
bodyweight, use of 80, 82
bouncing from foot to foot, as warning signal 35
breakaway techniques 78–105
    learning 76–8
    medical implications 78
    *see also specific techniques*
    personal space 72–6
breathing
    increased rate 35, 40
    reducing rate 40–1
    restriction 71
'broken record' principle 49, 60
'The Buck Passer' 63
bus travel 129–30

car maintenance 128
car travel 127–9
care plans 24
casualty departments 24, 134
catalysts *see* causative factors
causative factors 8–12
  case study 12–13
  clinical 14–17
  external 17–21
CCTV 24, 134
change, as causative factor
  medication 14
  routine 17
checking technique 45–7
choke/choking
  escaping from 92, 96, 98, 101
  rear 103–5
  *see also* neckholds
civil law 68
clenching and unclenching
    fists 36
clinical condition 14–17, 34
  mental health 12–13, 14,
    15, 16, 20
closed circuit television (CCTV)
    24, 134
clothing
  appropriate 55–6, 77, 126–7
  external risk management
    126–7
  grabs 90–5, 96–8, 99, 101–2
  learning practical techniques 77
cognitive abilities
  in confrontation 40
  in mental illness 12
colour
  code of awareness 25–6, 37
  of the face 35
communication 30–1, 44–7
  checking technique 45–7
  definition 58

of feelings and attitudes 45
  inability 14, 16
  the other perspective 48–50
  positive 58–61
  reasons for failure 58–60
  verbal confrontations 30, 31,
    43–4, 50–1, 64
  *see also* body language;
    information
community staff 5, 6–7,
    17–18, 19
  *see also* external causative
    factors; external risk
    management
compliant behaviour 30, 31
confidence
  appearance of 56–7
  determining 50–1
  eye contact 54–5
  knowledge and 41–2
conflict resolution plan 29–34, 37
  'extreme' needs 69–71
counsellors 118, 121
'The Counter Attacker' 63
Criminal Law Act (1967) 67

dark glasses 55
debriefing 117–18
  professionals 118, 119, 121
  timing of 119
delusional behaviour 16
departmental safety 133–5
diagonal wrist grab(s)
  control 84–6
  frontal 80–4
disciplinary interviews 61–3
disorientation 14
distance *see* personal space
double-handed clothing grabs
    96–8, 99
double-handed wrist grabs 86–90

drugs *see* medication
duty of care 21, 66, 70, 84

elbow strikes 103–4, 105
'element of surprise' 76–7
'emotional balance' 118–20
emotional effects, post-incident
    116, 117
empathy
  in debriefing 118
  the other perspective 48–9
employee protection 4, 66, 134
environment
  awareness of 23–5
  causative factors 8–9, 15
European Convention for
    Human Rights (2000) 4
'excessive force' 67–9
external causative factors 17–21
external risk management
  car travel 127–9
  journey planning 123–5, 125,
    127, 128
  personal alarms 131–3
  public transport 129–30
  walking 125–7
'extreme' needs 69–71
extreme violence *30*, 31
eye contact 54–5
  avoidance 28–9, 55
  maintaining in breakaway
    techniques *91*, *95*
  prolonged 35

facial colour 35
facial expression 54–5
factual information 60, 61, 64
'fake' body language 51
fatigue, as impact factor 33
fear *see* 'fight or flight'
feedback 60, 61

'fight or flight' 38–9
  physiology and effects 34–5,
    39–41
  'red' code 25–6
  understanding 41–2
  *see also* adrenalin
fingers, risk of injury 86, 90, 92,
    95, 96, 98, 102
fists, clenching and
    unclenching 36
freezing 41
frontal diagonal wrist
    grabs 80–6
frontal hair grab 98, *100*, 101
frontal straight-on wrist
    grab 79–80
frustration 12

'gap'
  'reactionary gap' 74, *101*
  in understanding 61–2
gestures 55
  hospitable 44–5
  'open' hands *52*, 73
'go' system *see* 'fight or flight'
grabs 75
  clothing 90–8, 99
  hair 98, *100*, 101
  shoulder 102–3
  wrist 79–90

hair grab, frontal 98, *100*, 101
hands
  encumbered 75
  'open' *52*, *73*, *88*, *89*
  position/movement 36, 55
  pulling 82
  shaking 56
head
  blows to 71
  position of 28–9, 53

Health and Safety at Work Act (1974) 4, 66, 134
heart rate, in confrontation 39–40
home safety 130–1
home visits 5, 128
    *see also* external causative factors; external risk management
hospitable gestures 44–5
humour 49

impact factors 31–4
inability to communicate 14, 16
inactivity, as causative factor 17
information
    communication of 50–1, 57–8
    factual 60, 61, 64
    lack of 10–11, 15
    repetition of 49, 60
    retention of 57–8
    *see also* communication; knowledge
'The Injured Innocent' 63
injury
    as impact factor 33
    risk of 71, 78
        *see also* joints; wrist
interviews 61–5
    arrangements 64, 65
    difficult interviewees 63–4
    interruptions 60
irrationality 20–1

jaw, facial expression 55
joints 69
    pain compliance controls 70, 106, 107, 109
    risk of injury 86, 90, 92, 95, 96, 98, 102, 111
journey planning 123–5, 127, 128, 134–5

keys
    car 128
    house 127, 130
knowledge 34, 41–2, 60
    *see also* information

lack of information 10–11, 15
lack of time 50, 59–60
learning *see* training
learning difficulties 12–13, 14, 15
legal actions 67–8
'The Legal Eagle' 63
legislation
    Criminal Law Act (1967) 67
    Health and Safety at Work Act (1974) 4, 66, 134
    Mental Health Act (1983) 71
lighting, movement-sensitive 131
listening 59, 60

malice 19
managers *see* interviews
medication
    changes in 14
    drugs and alcohol 20–1, 32
Mental Health Act (1983) 71
mental health issues 12–13, 14, 15, 16, 20
'minimum/reasonable force' 67, 68–9, 75
mobile phones *124, 125, 126,* 128
motives *see* causative factors
motor skills
    in confrontation 40
    in mental illness 12
mouth, facial expression 55
movement-sensitive lighting 131
'mugging' *see* theft

neckholds 71
*see also* choke/choking
NHS settings, incidence of
    aggression 1–3, 6–7
'no smoking' policy 9
'no-go' areas of the body 69–71
noradrenalin 34–5, 41, 118–19
note-taking 46
number of individuals, as impact
    factor 33

obsessions 16
'open' hands
    breakaway technique *88, 89*
    gesture *52*, 73
open questions 46, 47, 48, 59
'orange' code 25, 26
organization
    causative factors 9–10
    employee protection 4, 66, 134
    policy on self-defence 66–9, 84
the other perspective 48–50

pain
    as causative factor 16, 47
    compliance controls 70, 106,
        107, 109
panic buttons 24, 133
passiveness 28
perception, in confrontation 40
personal alarms 24, 131–3,
    134–5
personal disclosure 48–9, 118
personal gain *see* theft
personal possessions
    in car 127
    on person 127
Personal Safety Promotion (PSP)
    114, 117, 138, 139
personal space/distance 15, 54,
    72–6

physical interventions 106–12
physical size, as impact factor 32
physical strength, as impact
    factor 32
'positional asphyxia' 71
positive communication 58–61
positive psychotic symptoms 16
positive statements 48
post-incident
    case study 120, 121
    emotional effects 116, 117
    management 117–21
post-traumatic stress disorder
    (PTSD) 117
posture
    balanced and stable 74–5
    warning signals 35, 36, 53
proactive *vs* reactive strategies
    114–15
professional approach
    body language 53–7
    debriefing 118, 119, 121
'The Professional Weeper' 63
progression technique 111, *112*
PSP *see* Personal Safety
    Promotion
psychological effects, post-inci-
    dent 116, 117
psychotic symptoms, positive 16
PTSD *see* post-traumatic stress
    disorder
public transport 129–30

questions
    closed 46, 47
    open 46, 47, 48, 59

'reactionary gap' 74, *101*
reactive *vs* proactive strategies
    114–15
rear choke 103–5

rear shoulder grab 102–3
'reasonable/minimum force' 67, 68–9, 75
recovery position 71
'red' code 25–6
restoring 'emotional balance' 118–20
retention of information 57–8
'road rage' 127
routine, change in 17

screaming 132–3
secure units 133, 134
sensory faculties, in confrontation 40
sex, as impact factor 32
sexual assaults 19–20
shaking hands 56
shoulder
  rear grab 102–3
  risk of injury 86, 90, 92, 95, 96, 98, 102, 111
single-handed clothing grabs 90–5, 101
sitting down 44
size, as impact factor 32
skill level, as impact factor 33
smiling 54, 55
'spy holes' 131
staff attitudes 11, 28
stance see posture
staring 54–5
street crime see theft
strength, as impact factor 32
striking 70–1, 75, 102
  rear choke 103–4, 105
suffocation risk 71
'swan-neck' wrist lock 109, *110*

target locating, as warning signal 36
taxi travel 130

team mechanics 28
telephone
  listings/answering 130–1
  mobile 124, 125, 126, 128
  public 125
tension releasing technique 40–1
theft 18–19, 122–3, 125
time factors
  communication 50, 59–60
  debriefing 119
  visiting 'bad' neighbourhoods 124
  waiting times 10
tone of voice 27, 45, 55
train travel 130
training 5–6, 76–8, 137, 138
  courses 139
travel see external risk management

United Kingdom Central Council for Nursing, Midwifery and Health Visiting (UKCC) 6, 138

verbal confrontations 30, 31, 43–4, 50–1, 64
'vicarious liability' 68
visual aids 57, 61
visual contact see eye contact
voice, tone of 27, 45, 55
vulnerable position, as impact factor 33

waiting times, as causative factor 10
walking alone 125–7
ward safety 133–5
warning signals 34–7
weapons 32–3, 133
  potential 15, 75
'white' code 25, 26

'withdrawal statements' 46–7, 49
wrist
  grabs 79–90
  risk of injury 80, 84, 86, 90,
    92, 95, 96, 98, 102

'swan-neck' wrist lock 109,
  *110*
written information 57

'yellow' code 25, 26